The Body House
E. Margaret Lawrence

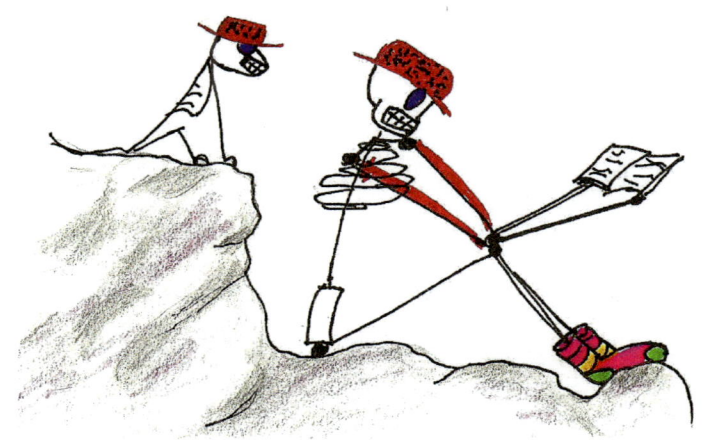

Copyright April 09, 2004 TXu1-176-941

ACKNOWLEDGEMENTS

Nothing is ever written without an inspiration from somewhere. The inspiration for this book was from "the body house" in which we live. The magnificence of structure and operation are awe-inspiring. Youth, the inheritors of our lives and civilization, have an insatiable curiosity about the bodies in which they live. This book is for them, an open door for exploration.

This idea, finally on paper, came to the attention of Leah Barnier. Leah saw where it should go, and sent it on its way. My eternal thanks to you, Leah.

I would also like to thank specific members of the medical profession who read the book and made valuable suggestions:

Doctors Pam Bundy, Paul Hoque, Robert Love, Stuart Nemir, Larry Campodonico, and to Gail Tate, PT, OCS.

FORWARD

No matter what kind, size or shape, the bodies of animal and man are masterpieces of life to be respected. They represent so many complexities of engineering, function and art that total understanding is yet to be accomplished. One who studies these masterpieces does so with awe, and wonder if this understanding will ever be fulfilled.

The human body is, by far, the most complex. Centuries have been consumed in study of all aspects of function, from artists who render duplications on canvass and in marble, to scientists who meticulously dissect from surface to miniscule, internal cell construction.

This book is dedicated to the magnificence of the human body. These words would not be on this page without the complex uses of parts of parts this intricate machine. In their own inevitable way, youngest of our species want to know the "what's" and "how's" of our Body House. The following story is meant take them by the "mental hand" and embark on a "body" trip, with their fearless leader "Ghost Host" and friends, Enod Ton and Eninac.

INVENTORY FOR CONSTRUCTION

WELCOME	*1*
1. FRAMING *SKELETON*	*3*
2. SIDING *MUSCLE*	*9*
3. CONVEYER SYSTEM *HEART AND CIRCULATION*	*13*
4. VENTILATION *RESPIRATION*	*19*
5. THE KITCHEN *DIGESTION*	*25*
HALF TIME	
6. ELECTRICAL SYSTEM *NERVOUS SYSTEM*	*31*
7. THE COMPUTER *BRAIN*	*43*
8. SENSORS *SENSES*	*49*
9. DUCTWORKS *GLANDS*	*59*
10. WATERPROOF BARRIER *SKIN*	*65*
DECISION TIME	*73*
AN END AND A BEGINNING	*75*

WELCOME

Ghost Host stood in front of the group of students in their classroom. The students could not see him, but they could hear him.

"Hello, Student Guests! Welcome to our adventure called THE BODY HOUSE. I am your Ghost Host. I will talk with you as we travel through THE BODY HOUSE but you will never see me. My friend, Enod Ton, is looking for the rest of his body, and I will help him find what he needs. You'll meet Enod Ton, and you can help make him (or her) a complete person. AH! Here he comes now!"

Ghost Host said, "Enod Ton, come and meet our guests."

Enod Ton clattered to the front of the room. "Hello, student guests. My name is Enod Ton. That name sounds strange, you might say. Let me give you a clue, read it backward. What does it say? RIGHT! Not Done. As you can see, I am missing a few dozen parts. If we work with Ghost Host, we can find the parts I need to make me a whole person. Ghost Host tells me we can find everything in THE BODY HOUSE."

Enod Ton moved closer to the students. "Am I a boy or a girl? I don't know yet. For now, I'll be a "he" but many things can change and you may be surprised. We can decide that together as we go through THE BODY HOUSE. Let's look at what I have right now. That way, we can see what's missing."

Enod Ton stood up and rattled off to look in a mirror. He shook his head and said to the students, "There's a lot missing. We have so much to do that I may need a short rest before we begin."

Ghost Host and Enod Ton sat down while the students chatted among themselves.

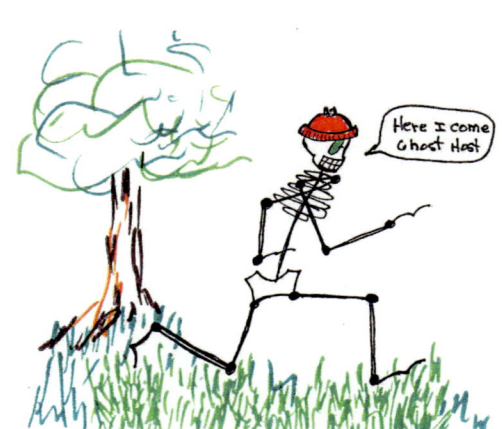

FRAMEWORK

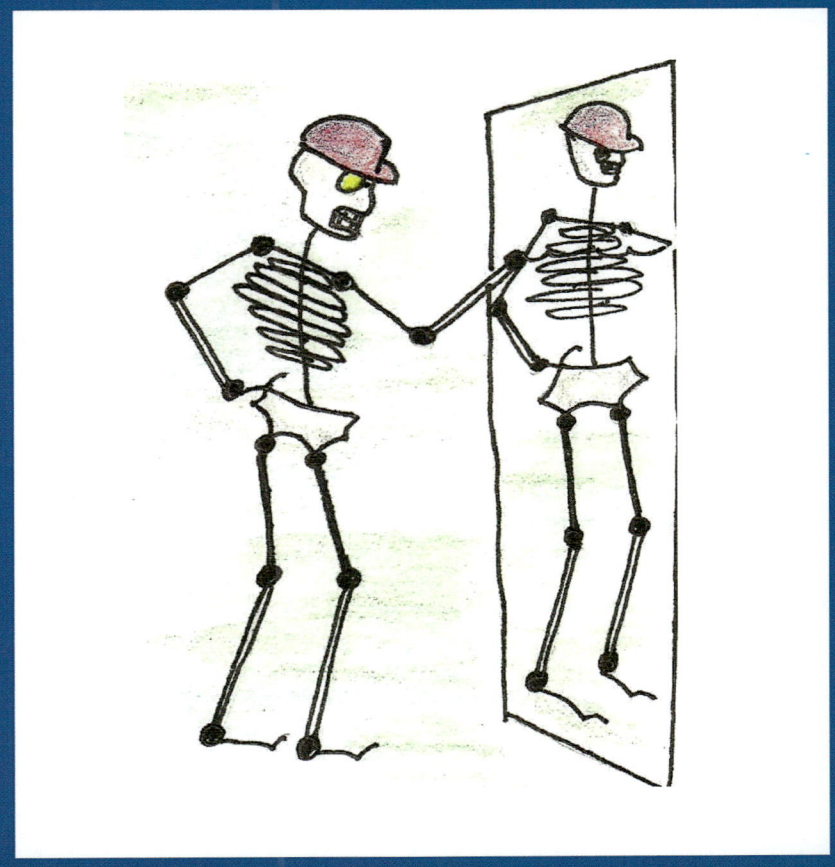

"The very first thing built for a house is the FRAMEWORK. The same is true of the body. Enod Ton, what is the framework of the body?"

Enod Ton looked around at the Student Guests, hoping for some help.

"They're not going to help you. Go look in the mirror. Tell me what you see."

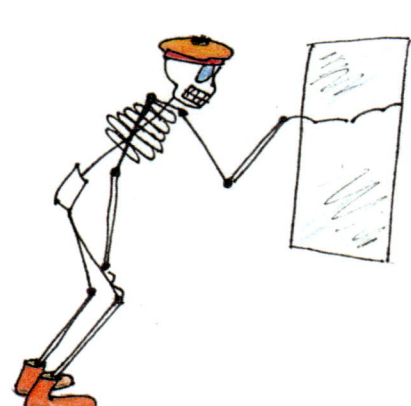

Enod Ton clattered over to the mirror. "Ghost Host, That's me! I know what I am! A SKELETON! That's my framework. I'm just like a house. With framework."

"Right. And from the way you look, you have a good-looking start for a fine body."

Enod Ton walked around in a circle, watching himself. "I am good looking, don't you think? Just look at how many bones I have. The shapes are all so different. Why is that, Ghost Host?"

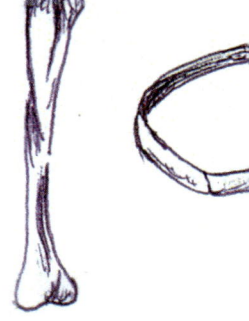

Ghost Host sighed. "All he has is bones and he thinks he's handsome. To answer your question, Enod Ton, you have straight bones like in your arms and curved bones like your ribs. One is even like a bowl. Do you know which one that is?"

Enod Ton stopped walking about and looked harder in the mirror. "Of course I know. It's my skull. I use my skull to wear my hats." Enod Ton smiled with pride, knowing he was right.

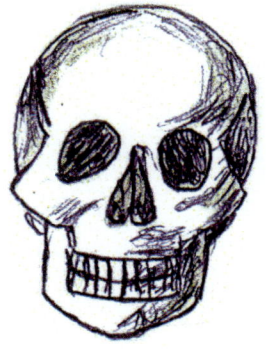

Ghost Host was trying to collect a few thoughts. "HATS! That's not the main job of the skull, Enod Ton. The skull holds and protects the brain."

"I knew that. Well, maybe I didn't. Right, Ghost Host. I forgot the brain. I'll wear hats anyway. My head-bone gets cold." Enod Ton smiled (we think!).

Ghost Host decided it was best to talk about what was next in the bone department.

"Tip your head forward and feel the back of your neck. What are the ridges you feel? Neck bones? Right. They are called vertebrae. They go all the way down your back. The official name for them is the vertebral column."

Enod Ton was still feeling the bones of his neck and back. "There are so many different shapes. Even the vertebrae are different. Why is this, Ghost Host?"

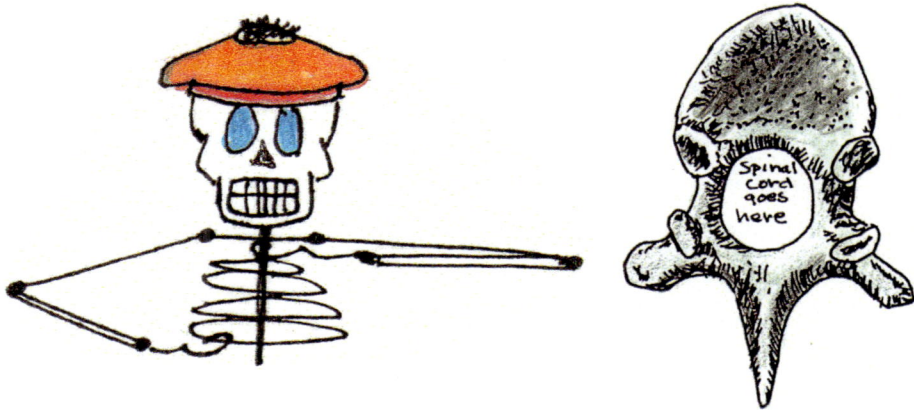

"Good Question, Enod Ton. The vertebrae do two things. They let you stand up straight. (All parents say, "Stand up straight"). The second thing is to hold and protect the communication system of the body, called the spinal cord. "

"How exciting! Is my body going to communicate with something?"

"You are constantly communicating with everything around you. Your brain sends messages all over your body, Enod Ton. They travel through the spinal cord, and that is the body's communication system. We will talk more about that later."

Enod Ton was thinking about the bones. "Bones don't bend, Ghost Host. How can I take dancing lessons?"

"Glad you asked. There are special pads between the vertebrae made of cartilage. It is smooth and a bit spongy. This lets you move in many directions without breaking the bones. This same cartilage is on the ends of most all of your bones. This lets you move smoothly."

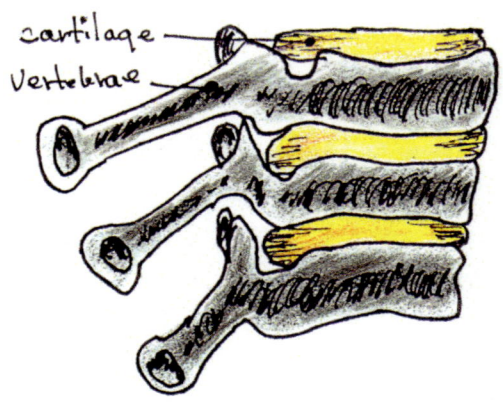

Enod Ton tried dancing a few steps. "HA! It works - just like you said. I would like learning the Tango." As he danced by the student guests, he stopped, watched how they were writing. "Hands are wonderful things, Ghost Host. Look at how our guests are holding pencils and writing things."

"Hands are certainly wonderful, Enod Ton. They can do so many things. They also hold cookies while you're eating them."

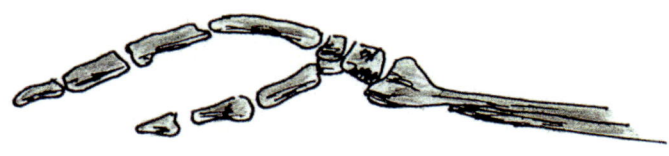
That got Enod Ton's attention immediately. "What a grand idea. I will make tea to go with the cookies, and help you at the same time." While Enod Ton was preparing tea and cookies, Ghost Host was preparing another bone-story.

"Let's talk about the "longest and the strongest". There is a bone in your body that's both of those. It connects your hips with your knees and it even has a name. It is called the femur." Ghost Host suddenly had an idea. "I'll sing a bone song."

Enod Ton was smiling (but no one knew that) because Ghost Host was singing off key.

Ghost Host ended the song on a long high note. "There. That should tell you enough about bones. If Enod Ton has finished his cookies and tea, (and the dishes) I would like to tell you about joints."

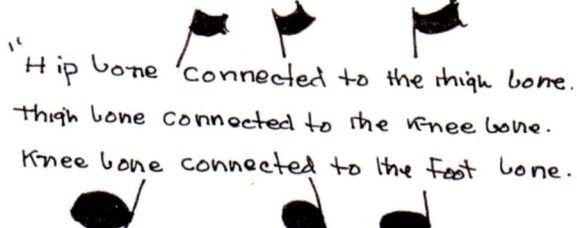

Enod Ton was just finishing, and hurried to join Ghost Host.
"While you were singing ten verses about bones, I was looking up bone joints in your book. There are four kinds and I shall be glad to explain them all."

Ghost Host was very surprised. "Good gracious, Enod Ton. Please do explain about joints." Ghost Host sat down (we think) to listen.

"Student Guests, pay close attention and follow directions. Let's start at the top of your body, which I have discovered is the head. "Enod Ton patted the top of his golf hat. "Turn your head from side to side, now up and down, now in circles. Why can you do this? Because the neck is a **pivot** joint."

Ghost Host was following the directions. At least, we think so. "Enod Ton that was a very good explanation. I did those exercises, too. "(Aha! We thought so). "Would you like for me to continue?"

"Oh no, I am rolling along fine. Now look at your elbow. You can straighten your arm but only so far. That is called a **hinge** joint. There is another hinge joint. Do you know where it is? Right, Your knees! Your ankles and wrists are **gliding** joints because they move in many directions.

"Enod Ton is right. The last joint is my favorite. It is the **ball and socket** joint. Student guests stand up and pretend that you are throwing a ball. See how your arm can go around in a circle? Your legs can move in kind of a circle, too. That is because your arms, and your hips have ball and socket joints."

Enod Ton was still swinging his arms. He even danced a few steps so that he could watch his hip joints. "I certainly do understand a lot more about bones and joints. I have a fine framework for the rest of my body. I shall be very handsome - even more than I am now."

Ghost Host was listening to Enod Ton's discussion with himself. "What is handsome about all of those bare bones? I will admit that I like his hats. Those are handsome. His socks are terrible."

"Ghost Host, I must go to the library and get some books. Yours don't have enough information. I may pick up a cookie cookbook, too."

Off they went in Ghost Host's rusty little car. No one knew what kind it was because the name had fallen off.

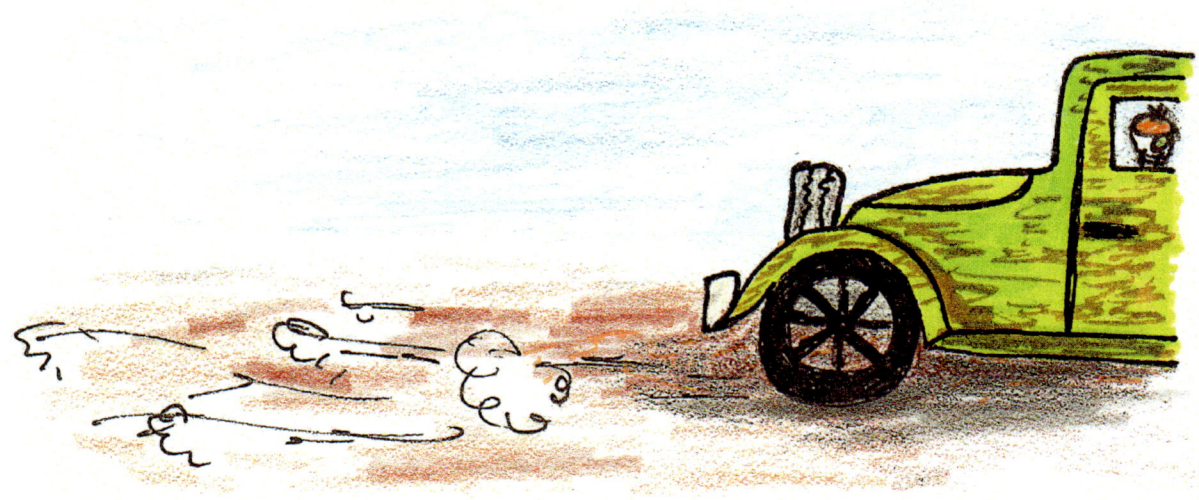

SIDING

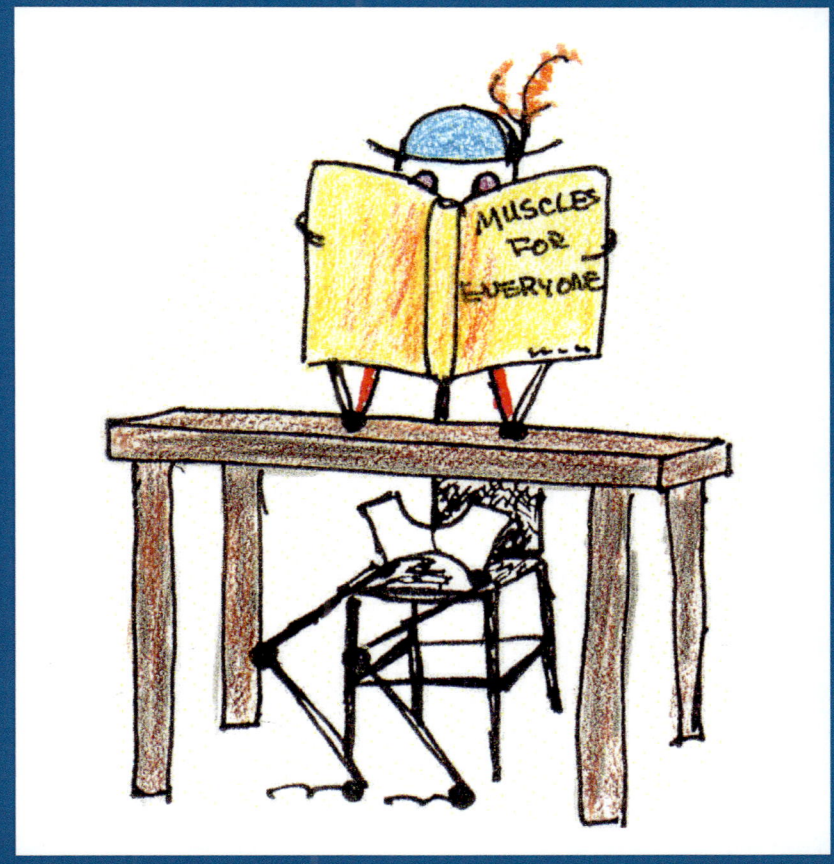

Our next step for Enod Ton is **SIDING**. We can't let him walk around looking like a Halloween leftover. Enod Ton's bony body needs shape. How can we do this? With muscle. Muscle gives the body its shape.

Now to add muscle to the bones. In our BODY HOUSE construction, we have to connect the muscles to the bones. White glue will not work. Wire? Enod Ton may not like that. Enod Ton, would you like to give us some information about muscle attachment?

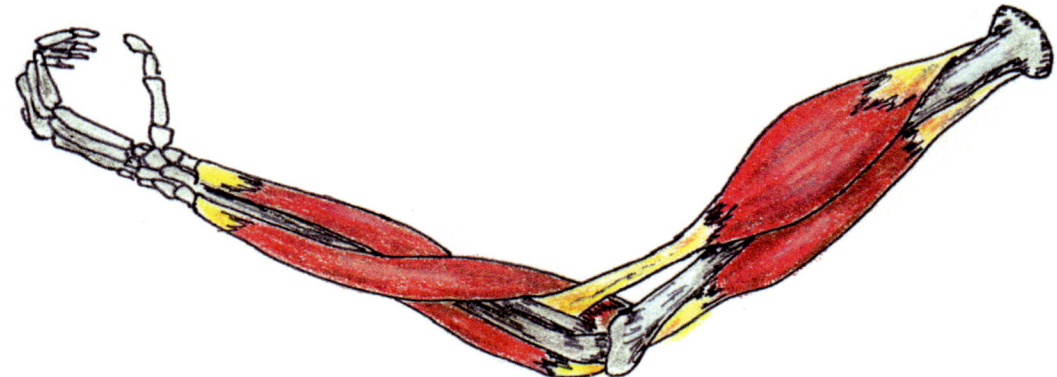

"I will be happy to, if you promise not to use wire. Muscles are attached to the bones with tendons. All muscles on the skeleton have tendons at each end of the muscle. The tendons have special cells which grow to the bones and hold the muscle tight to the ends of the bone."

This type of muscle is called SKELETAL muscle because it is attached to the skeleton. That makes sense. The more you use it, the stronger it gets. If muscles are not used for even a short a period of time, they get smaller and weaker. Muscles used often and well, have what we call good muscle tone.

"Use it or loose it," said Enod Ton.

That's true, Enod Ton. Let's look further into that idea. Stand up, Student Guest. That simple action set in motion thousands of complex activities. To stand up, you used almost every skeletal muscle you have. If Enod Ton has finished his tea, perhaps he will help us with muscles and moving.

Enod Ton had finished his tea and was reading one of his many catalogs, shopping for person-parts. He wanted to make sure what he was looking for was the right thing.

Enod Ton, could you please explain to our guests how and why they could stand up?

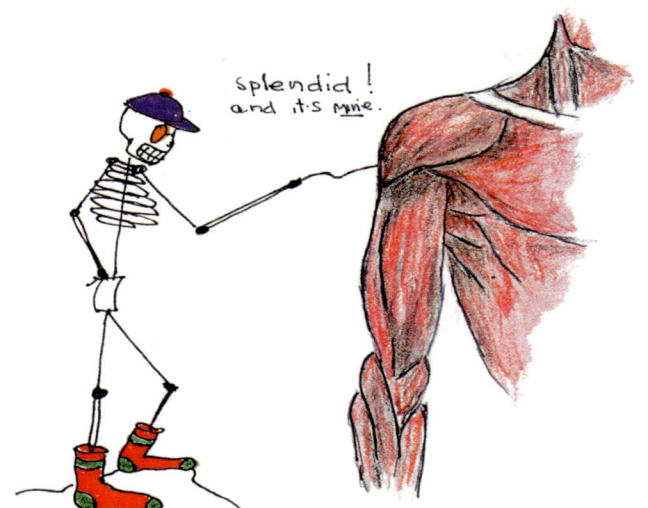

"Hold on, just a moment. Here is a part called gluteus maximus. I may need that. Now, how and why did you stand up? In every muscle, no matter how small, large or which type, there are nerves. Ghost Host asked you to stand up. Your brain picked up the message, sent it over the nerves to your muscles. Your muscles did their job of contracting and expanding, and you stood up. Later, your visit will take you to the communications department and you will learn how this message travels. Right now, I need to have you help me get into shape."

"OK, Student Guests, while Enod Ton is looking at muscles that go on his skeleton, let's look at how a muscle lives. Did you know that muscles must be fed? Yes, they need food. How and what do they eat? Your muscles "eat" what you eat. If you have a good diet of necessary foods, your muscles will prosper and get rich. They also need oxygen. Muscles have lungs? No, but you do. What you inhale goes to all parts of your body, including your muscles. We will look further into that when we get to the Ventilation System.

Let me give you another example of how oxygen works in your muscles. Do you see that goal post down on the playing field? Run down there and back. That was a fast run- but you are breathing more rapidly and heavier than before. This is because your muscles need more oxygen to move faster and harder. When you breathe more rapidly after running, your muscles have oxygen debt. You owe your muscles more oxygen and you will breathe like this until all of the oxygen is returned to your muscles. Sometimes, after you have used your muscles more than usual, they feel sore and it hurts a bit to move."

Enod Ton is still looking at his catalog. "Aha! Blue hair? Err, no, I don't think so. Sore muscles? I don't have any yet but I will tell you what happens. Using your muscles in normal, everyday activity causes normal, everyday muscle waste to form. Your body has its own trash pick-up, and it does this constantly.

When you are unusually active, your muscles create more waste and the body takes longer to remove it. The waste is called lactic acid. The lactic acid irritates the muscles until it is picked up in one or two days. There is no damage to your muscles, but this can be prevented by slowly conditioning your muscles to more vigorous activity."

"That was a good explanation, Enod Ton. We already know that the muscles just under the skin are called skeletal muscles. We can see their shape. There are two other kinds of muscles we cannot see. They are inside our bodies. **Cardiac** muscle is found in only one place in our bodies. Do you know where?"

Enod Ton looked up from his catalog. "It is the heart muscle. It never stops working."

Right! It contracts about 80 times a minute, all day and night, every day and night. Even holidays. We will get to know our heart when we visit the "conveyer system" of the BODY HOUSE.

The last kind of muscle we have is called **smooth** muscle. It makes your internal organs work automatically. It pushes your blood through your blood vessels, moves the food along your digestive road, and does dozens of other jobs. Your brain runs smooth muscle and cardiac muscle automatically. Skeletal muscle is mostly under your control. You tell it what to do."

Enod Ton was smiling (we think). He was anxious to explain something. "Ghost Host, I'll bet you are still wondering why I need gluteus maximus muscles. Our guests already have them and they use them a lot. Student Guests, you are all sitting down. You are sitting on them!"

CONVEYER SYSTEM

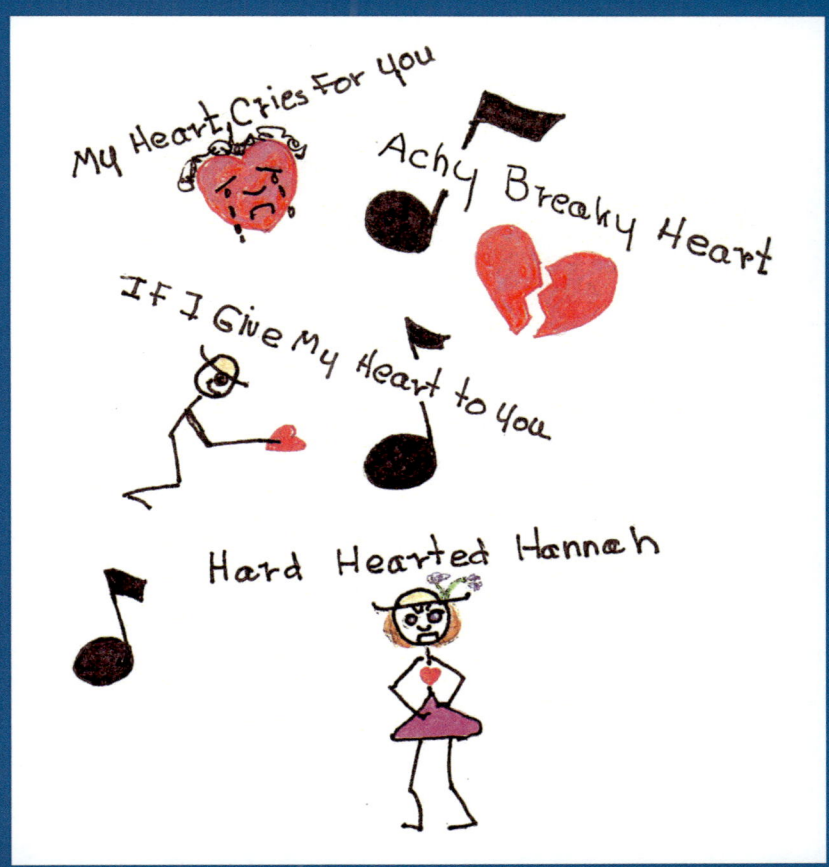

The body has a subway called the **CONVEYER SYSTEM**. It might also be referred to as "the heart of the matter".

"Ghost Host, I have found the heart of the matter." said Enod Ton as he raced up the steps to the library, looking for his friend.

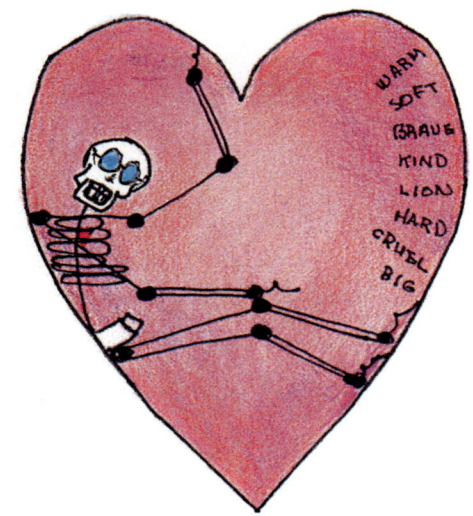

Enod Ton is still rattling as he moves because he does not have all of his muscles yet. Ghost Host heard him coming.

I am in here, Enod Ton. I hope that you get something on those bones soon. You are very noisy. What and where is the "heart of the matter"?

Enod Ton dropped onto a chair and said. "The heart of the matter is I have a heart! I know how the Tin Man in THE WIZARD OF OZ felt after he got his heart. Now I can sing all of those old songs about hearts and know what they mean."

Ghost Host liked the idea and immediately began singing in a slightly off-key voice.

Enod Ton listened to a few of the songs and said, "If you love something, is it your heart that loves it?"

No. Your heart has only one job to do and that is to pump blood to all areas of your body. Your brain controls everything your heart does. When your brain gives it a signal, your heart will beat faster or harder. Since your heart is a pump, lets go back to our song titles. Substitute the word "pump" for heart.

Try this one. My Heart Cries For You. Now, My Pump Cries For You. HA!

"That gives me a whole new way to think about a heart. I know what a heart looks like." said Enod Ton. "It looks like a valentine."

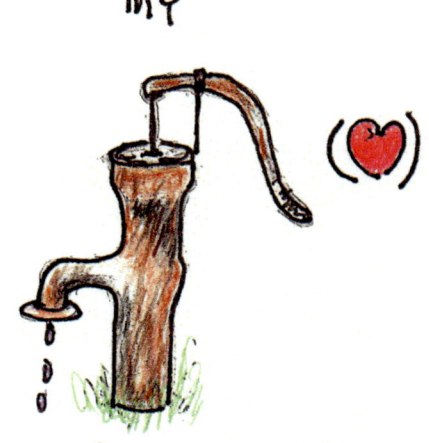

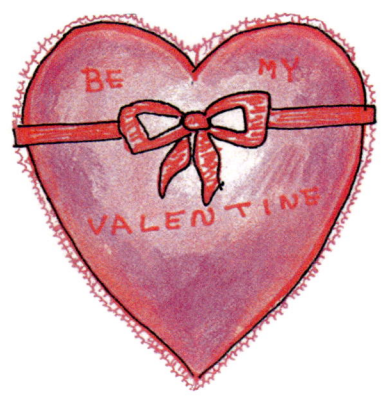

Ghost Host felt that rescue was necessary at this point. That makes a nice picture but your heart does not really look like that. Look at my picture of a heart and you will get a better idea of how it works.

In this drawing you can see that a heart has two sides and a top and bottom. Each part of your heart has a name and a special job to do. If you will look at the second drawing of a heart, you will see lines going in several directions. Follow the lines and you will see what each part of the heart does.

Enod Ton looked at the drawings and shook his head. "It looks like I really have two hearts."

Ghost Host looked at Enod Ton in amazement. A wonderful observation, Enod Ton. Although you really only have one heart, it does two jobs. It is an amazing organ. It never stops pumping blood to all parts of the body. This is what we call a heartbeat.

Enod Ton thought about all of this; then said, "But how does the blood get to where it is supposed to go?"

Ghost Host jumped up on the chair, arms swinging like an orchestra conductor. This is a very exciting part, Enod Ton. From this side of the heart the blood is squeezed out to your body. It travels through tubes called arteries. The arteries are large when they leave the heart and get smaller and smaller until they become tiny. When they are the smallest, they change to veins. The veins get larger and larger and carry the blood back to the heart.

Enod Ton looked at the drawing again and said, "That is amazing!"

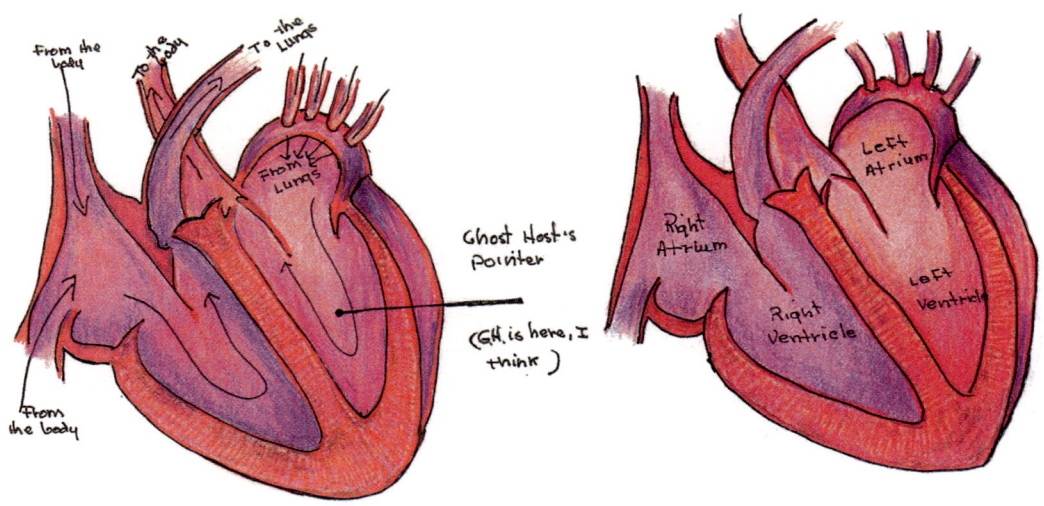

Ghost Host was still excited. That's not all, Enod Ton. The blood is the delivery service of the body. It picks up oxygen from the lungs. It picks up digested food from the small intestine. It delivers all of this to each and every cell in the body. Every cell needs both food and oxygen, and the blood delivers to the cell's front door, just like mail delivery.

Enod Ton was still thinking about arteries and what they do. Then he remembered another word; vein.

"There was another part you mentioned. It was called vein," said Enod Ton.

Ghost Host was still standing on the chair, waving the pointer. My friend, you are keeping me on track. Yes, the veins. Just as your cells need food and oxygen to live, they also have waste they need to send away. As the fresh blood passes through the body we know it delivers food and oxygen. As it starts back toward the heart, it picks up waste materials. These are carried off to other areas of the body to be disposed of.

"Well now that is something else!" said Enod Ton. "There must be several feet of arteries and veins."

Ghost Host muttered loudly about I thought you would never ask. Oh yes, we do have several feet as you mentioned, however, let's talk about miles. An adult has about 100,000 miles of arteries and veins.

This was too much for Enod Ton. He stood up and looked at Ghost Host. "But I don't have room in my body for all of that. Look at this. Where is it all going to go?"

Ghost Host got down off the chair, sat down and tried to calm Enod Ton. Oh yes, it will all fit. Not only that, there are many other things to go into your body which we have not even discussed yet.

There is one more thing that we had better mention. Do you think that you can handle this Enod Ton?

"I don't know. This has been so interesting, but there is so much to the body! YES! I can handle it all. Let's go on."

Ghost Host began the "blood story" with the red blood cells. They are what give your blood the red color, Enod Ton. These red cells are shaped like small saucers and are called corpuscles. The corpuscles carry the food and oxygen to feed all of the cells, everywhere in the body. The white blood cells are like the defending army of the body. If you get a splinter in your finger and don't remove it right away, it will become infected. The white material, which forms around the splinter, is made up of white blood cells, fighting the infection caused by the splinter.

Enod Ton's amazement increased. "An army to fight infection. Unbelievable!"

That's our **CONVEYER SYSTEM** story, Enod Ton. There are other parts that make up your blood. I think that you should look up some of these things while you are in the library. Let me add to your "look-up" list; what is a bruise and what are vein cups?

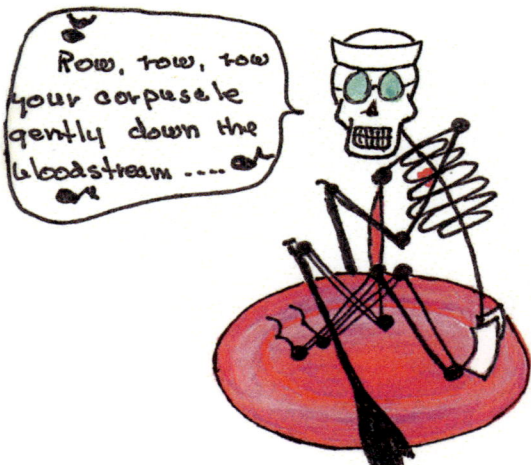

"Vein cups?" Enod Ton liked the idea of having an assignment. He said "I need to spend more time in the library, reading about what I have learned. While I am reading, I will look a little ahead for a "sneak preview" of what is to come"

VENTILATION SYSTEM

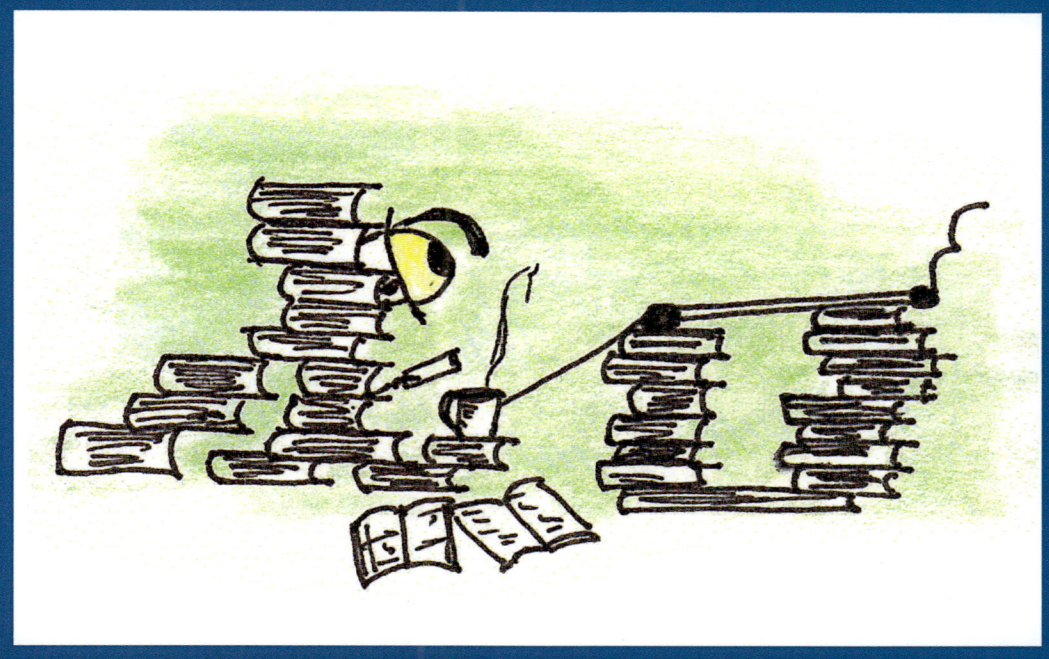

All houses need a **VENTILATION SYSTEM**. Our BODY HOUSE needs ventilation too. In the chapter on the blood, we discussed how blood carries oxygen. In this chapter we will talk more about that and other interesting things - like what makes it possible for you talk to your friends?

Enod Ton was just leaving the library when he saw Ghost Host getting in the car. "Wait, wait, Ghost Host! You can't leave now. We have too much to do." He ran down the steps to the street, arms loaded with books.

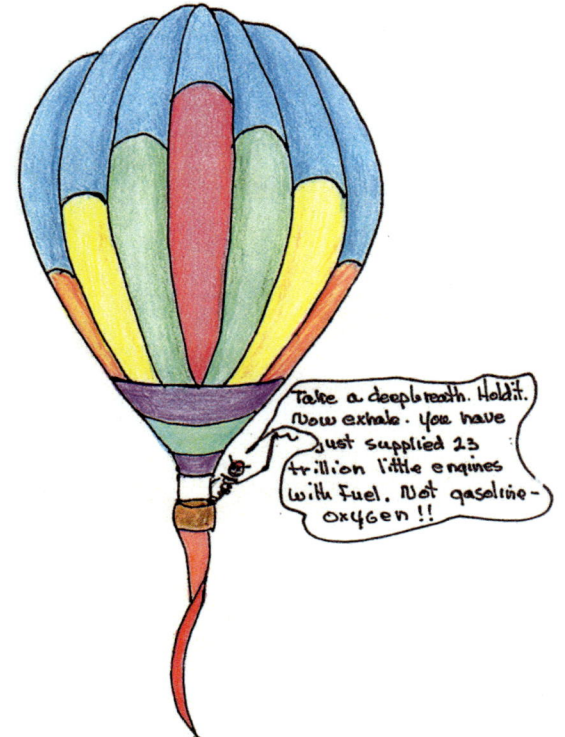

I am starving, Enod Ton. Ghosts have lunch once or twice a day. Get into the car and come with me.

Enod Ton rattled and banged getting into the car, books falling every which way.

Ghost Host saw all of the books. Did you leave any books in the library for the other students?

"Well, yes, a few." said Enod Ton. "Just look at what I found about the ventilation system and oxygen and fish and air sacs and earthworms and -------."

Whoa, Enod Ton. You ARE carried away. Good! Let's find a quick snack then look at what you have discovered.

After lunch, they found a quiet spot on the grass. Now, Enod Ton let's look at the way our bodies are ventilated. This is called breathing. The air enters your nose and --

"Yes! Quite right, Ghost Host!" said Enod Ton. "As the air goes down a long tube called the wind pipe or trachea, it is warmed to the temperature of your body and the dust is filtered out of it."

Enod Ton grinned (as much as possible) and watched, as Ghost Host's eyes got bigger. That's right, Enod Ton. Let's follow the trachea and see where it goes. There we are. It goes to the lungs.

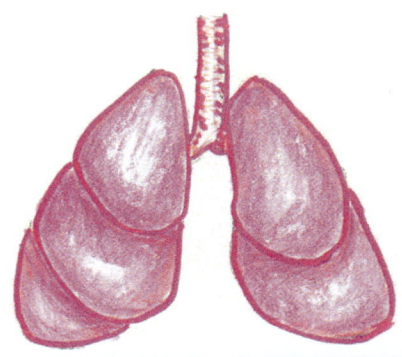

Enod Ton watched carefully and asked. "Why is the left lung smaller than the right lung?"

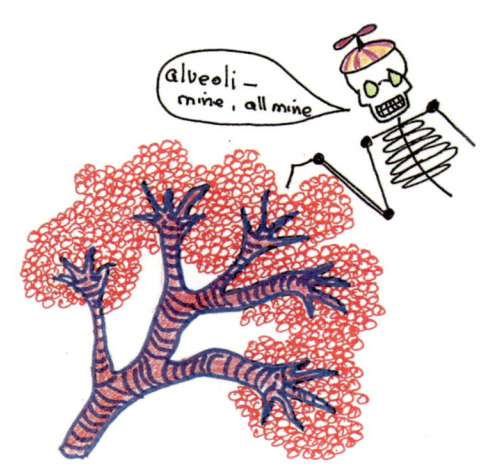

You noticed that, did you? Good observation. The left lung is smaller because your heart lives next to your left lung.

Enod Ton thought he would fool Ghost Host. "So, Ghost Host, if my heart is next to my left lung, does my left lung fall in love when my heart does?" Enod Ton thought to himself about what he had said, then muttered, half to himself, "Of course it doesn't!"

Ghost Host's eyes rolled around. You are too much, Enod Ton. Ghost Host was secretly laughing.

Since you have been reading and studying, Enod Ton, answer this. Are the lungs hollow bags?

"Oh no." said Enod Ton. "Lungs have tiny air sacs called alveoli everywhere inside them. Alveoli look like a sponge. When you take a breath these tiny sacs fill with air and bring oxygen into the lungs. When you breathe out, they squeeze together to force the carbon dioxide out of your body. "

Ghost Host could hardly wait for Enod Ton to finish his description of the alveoli. Now, Enod Ton, it is time to put some of our information together. Ghost Host stood up and said in a grand, deep voice, Enod Ton, remember how the blood goes to your lungs after it has been all over your body?

Why does it do that?

Enod Ton rattled to his feet, brushed the grass from his knee bones and said, "I know, exactly why that happens. When the blood comes back from traveling all over the body it has picked up waste and is not as clean as it was. It is dark red." He looked at Ghost Host to see if his teacher was following what he said.

Ghost Host smiled secretly and thought, he really knows what he is talking about. I must be an excellent teacher. Go on Enod Ton.

With much excitement, Enod Ton walked about, scattering books and papers, and continued his lesson. "The right side of the heart pumps the blood to the lungs where the waste material, called carbon dioxide, is exchanged for the clean oxygen. If you really think about it, Ghost Host, the lungs are a 'laundry' for the blood."

- larynx -
front on
trachea

Enod Ton was so pleased with his new idea, that the lungs are a "laundry", he hugged himself, then he did several dance steps.

Ghost Host was totally pleased. YES! That is the way it works. That is the way all of the parts of THE BODY HOUSE work - together!

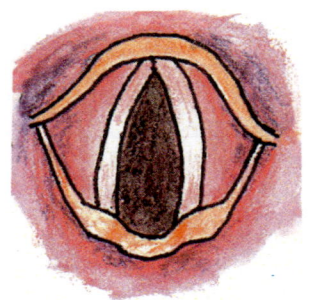
- Larynx - looking at vocal cords from the top.

The two of them sat down again. They were still excited but they knew that there were several important things necessary for even more understanding. Ghost Host took a deep breath then said, how do you know I am talking to you?

Enod Ton looked at Ghost Host with surprise. "I can hear your voice."

Before Ghost Host could say anything, Enod Ton said, "Wait! I know how it works - I know! "

Ghost Host said; well let's hear about it.

Enod Ton got to his feet, put his bony fingers on his neck and explained.

"In our wind pipe or trachea (as we learned to call it) there is a voice box called a larynx. You can feel it on your throat, under your chin. When we breathe, the air goes through it. There are two cords that go across the top of the larynx. These are called vocal cords. They are a little like guitar strings. When you talk, they vibrate."

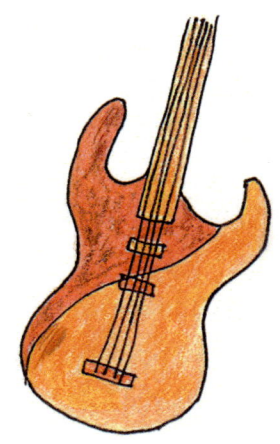

Ghost Host was following Enod Ton's vocal cord story carefully. You are right, Enod Ton. Let's try a little something. Put your hand on your throat, now say "AHHH". Do you feel the vibrations? Those are your vocal cords at work, vibrating.

Enod Ton thought for a moment then said, "One more thing to try, Ghost Host. Do you talk when you breathe in or out? Out, of course. Try to talk when you breathe in. It does not work too well, does it? Talking is done when you breathe out."

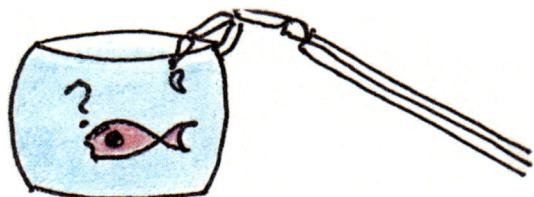

Ghost Host could hardly wait to ask Enod Ton more questions. Enod Ton, let go of your neck and answer more questions. How does a fish breathe? An earthworm? A grasshopper?

Back to the library and find out. Now wait a minute. I saw those questions answered in one of the Enod Ton stood very still and looked at Ghost Host. "Oh dear! I don't know. I must go library books."

Don't worry, Enod Ton, I shall tell you the answers. A fish breathes through its gills, an earthworm through its skin, and a grasshopper through slits in its abdomen called spiracles. How about that, Enod Ton?

"Fascinating! I must look up spiracles. Now I have a question for you, Ghost Host. Why do you have a hard time breathing when you are high in the air, on a high mountain?"

Ghost Host liked the idea of Enod Ton asking him questions.

Let me pretend to think a moment, and then I will ask, is it because there is not enough oxygen in the air at high altitude?

"Yes, Ghost Host, your answer is correct. I am proud of you, "said Enod Ton.

They both sat down and thought of all of the things they had discovered in the VENTILATION part of the BODY HOUSE. There were lungs, trachea, alveoli, larynx and how an earthworm breathes. Both Enod Ton and Ghost Host knew that they would use those, and more as they built Enod Ton a body.

Enod Ton, I am hungry.
Enod Ton looked at Ghost Host and said "Not again!"
Let's find a snack bar.

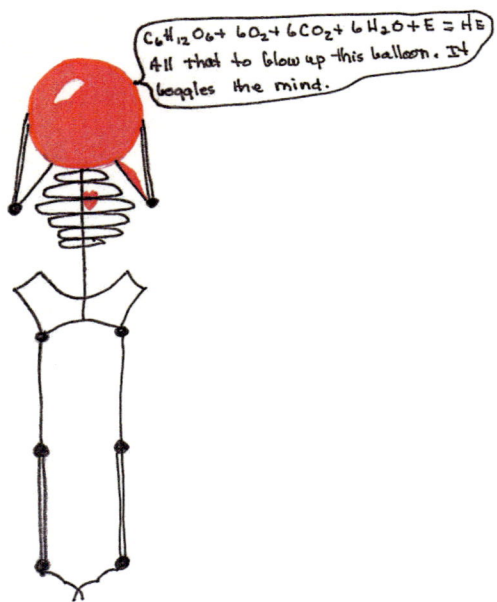

$C_6H_{12}O_6 + 6O_2 + 6CO_2 + 6H_2O + E = HE$
All that to blow up this balloon. It boggles the mind.

KITCHEN

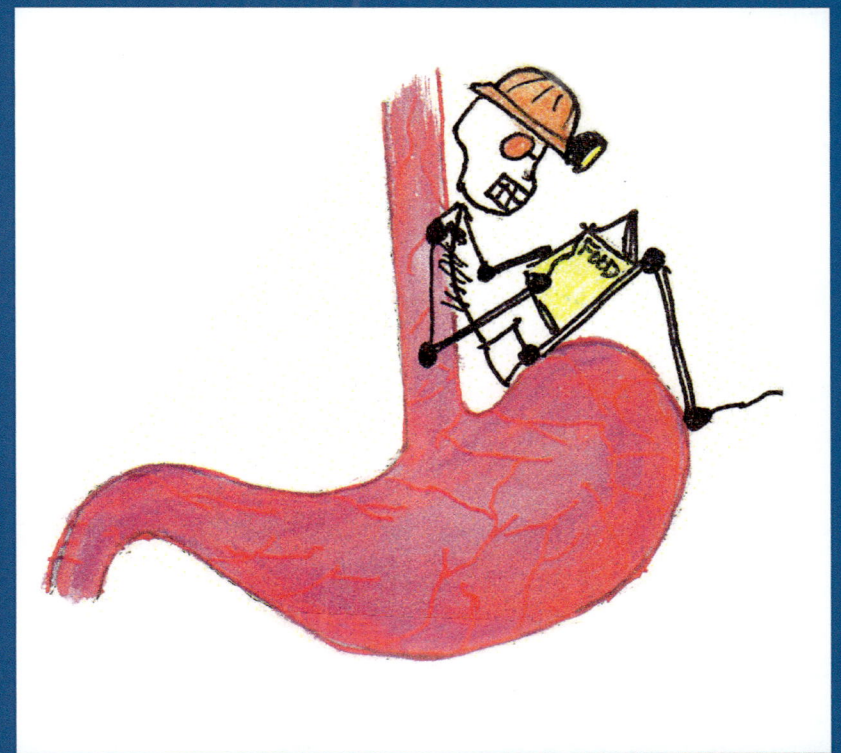

In every house there is **THE KITCHEN**. This is Ghost Host's favorite place in the whole house. He is about to be fooled because this kitchen does not cook anything. It takes care of the food after it is cooked.

Enod Ton was still surprised that Ghost Host was hungry again. "I can't understand why you are hungry so soon, Ghost Host. You do eat a lot."

Enod Ton, working with you keeps me hungry and thin. Just wait until you get your whole body. You will probably eat just for the fun of knowing what happens to your lunch after you have eaten it.

Enod Ton thought about this for a moment. "That might be true. Let me see, you had a sandwich and a glass of lemonade for lunch. Ghost Host, I have a glorious idea. Let's follow your lunch through your body and see what happens to it."

Ghost Host thought this was a spectacular idea. Where are your books, Enod Ton? They may be helpful.

As Enod Ton scurried after his scattered books he shouted, "Ghost Host, you do know that your 'body kitchen' does not cook anything."

Ghost Host's eyes rolled around. Thanks for telling me, Enod Ton. I would never have guessed. Then Ghost Host muttered -of course I knew that.

The two of them trotted off to a park bench and sat down. Enod Ton's books fell in every direction. He looked through the messy pile of books and found the one titled DIGESTION.

"A Ha, here it is. Now I'm ready to track your lunch, Ghost Host." Enod Ton opened the book and said, "Just ask me where digestion starts. No, don't. I'll tell you. It starts in the mouth."

True, Enod Ton. Since you are becoming an authority on the body you don't have yet, how did I know what I was tasting?

Enod Ton smiled and said, "I do know that. There are cells, called taste buds, in your mouth. Your tongue has these taste buds. Some buds taste salt, some sweet, some bitter and some sour. Here is a picture of where the taste buds are."

That's right, Enod Ton. When you chew, the water in your mouth, called saliva, mixes with the food. This makes the taste buds work. Did you know that if your mouth is dry you couldn't taste the food?

"No! Oh dear. I shall have to keep my mouth full of water all of the time."

You won't have to do that. There are glands in your mouth that make the saliva. When you eat something, they get to work and give your mouth the moisture it needs.

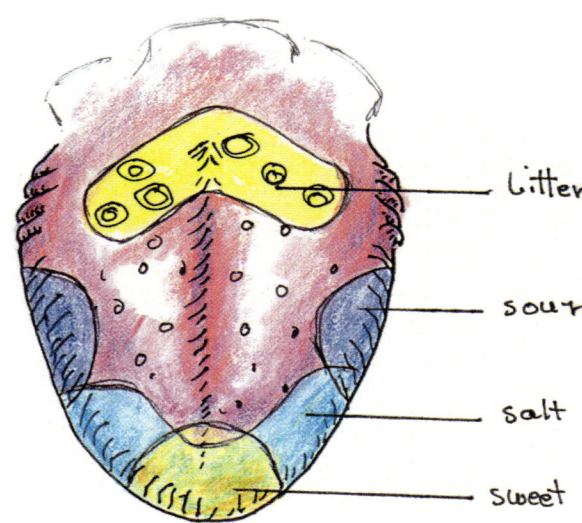

"Good arrangement. " said Enod Ton.

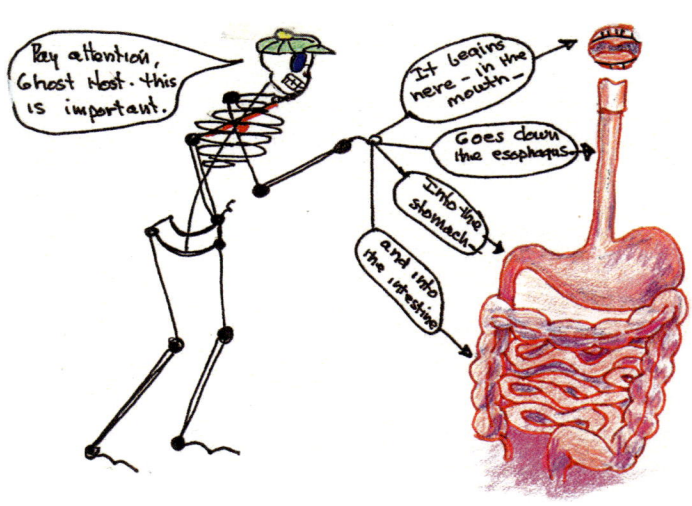

Ghost Host bit into a sardine sandwich as Enod Ton watched with great concentration. "How can I see what you and your sandwich are doing? You are almost always invisible. All I can hear is munch, munch."

Just watch the sandwich disappear, and you will know how my lunch is doing. You are sitting on a dozen books, Enod Ton. If you look for the one with details about digestion, you will have a good idea of what is happening.

Enod Ton rolled off the books to sit on the bench. He scrabbled through the pile until he found what he needed. "Don't eat too fast, Ghost Host.

I have to find the picture of the whole digestive route your sandwich will take. Here it is! OK, I'm ready."

Ghost Host was still munching. I am impressed with your explanation. This is a good sandwich. Maybe I'll have another one.

Enod Ton couldn't believe it. How can you eat so much Ghost Host? "I'm not really sure but I don't think you are very big.

When you get a stomach you will know how it feels. I might ask you, how much does a stomach hold?

Enod ton flipped through the pages of his book. "Whoa! I don't believe it. A stomach holds between 1 and 2 quarts. Quarts, Ghost Host. A stomach is a surprising organ."

Ghost Host smiled an I-knew-it all-the-time smile. Here's another question Enod Ton. We know that food moves through the body from mouth to waste department. How does it move?

"Gravity, of course." said Enod Ton.

Really, Enod Ton. Gravity! Tch,Tch. Let me explain. All of the organs where digestion takes place have muscles. These muscles are not like the ones you have on your arms and legs. These are specialized for moving food along the digestive tract. They are called smooth muscles. They work by squeezing and pushing the food along. This action is called peristalsis. Everything you eat moves through your body by peristalsis.

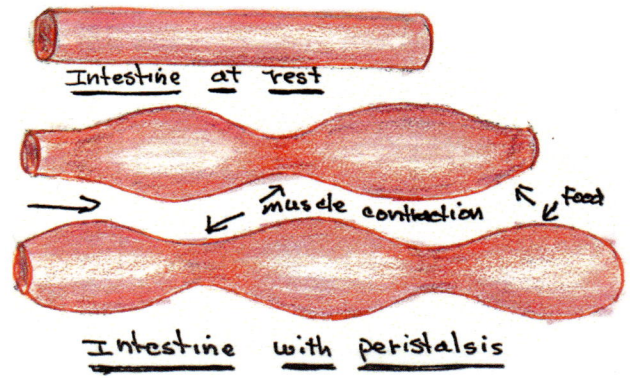

Enod Ton was so excited he thought about taking his sunglasses off. "Then everything we eat gets squeezed through all of those organs I showed you.

Your sandwich is getting squeezed now. Where is that sandwich?"

Ghost Host looked at the clock in the library tower. By now that sandwich should be in my small intestine.

Enod Ton was still sitting on the bench. He stood up with book in hand. "Ghost Host, I will tell you what is happening. As the food gets into the small intestine (look at the picture and you will see where the small intestine is), the intestine takes all of the good things like protein and iron and calcium out of the food as it goes through."

Right, Enod Ton. Do you know how long the small intestine is?

Enod Ton's sunglasses were still on but slightly askew. He flipped two pages. "This is unbelievable. In an adult, the small intestine is 20 to 22 feet. That long!"

Ghost Host was almost impressed himself. Your whole digestive tract is about 5 times as long as your body.

Enod Ton was trying to practice being "cool". "Of course, Ghost Host." He lost the "cool". "Five times? I am still thinking about where all of this is going to be put in my body."

Not to worry, Enod Ton. It will fit. We have more to talk about. After the food goes through the small intestine, it enters the large intestine. By now, all of the good parts of the food have been taken out by the small intestine. All we have left is waste. The large intestine takes out most of the liquid. It is preparing the waste for the body to get rid of it. The body moves the waste out about once a day.

Enod Ton was exhausted. "I need a rest after all of that. A body has so much. When I get all of my parts, I will have to take good care of them. "

Ghost Host was stretched out on the grass. Let's take a short nap, Enod Ton. If you had skin, you would have a tired look. Fix your sunglasses. We have a lot more to learn.

ELECTRICAL SYSTEM

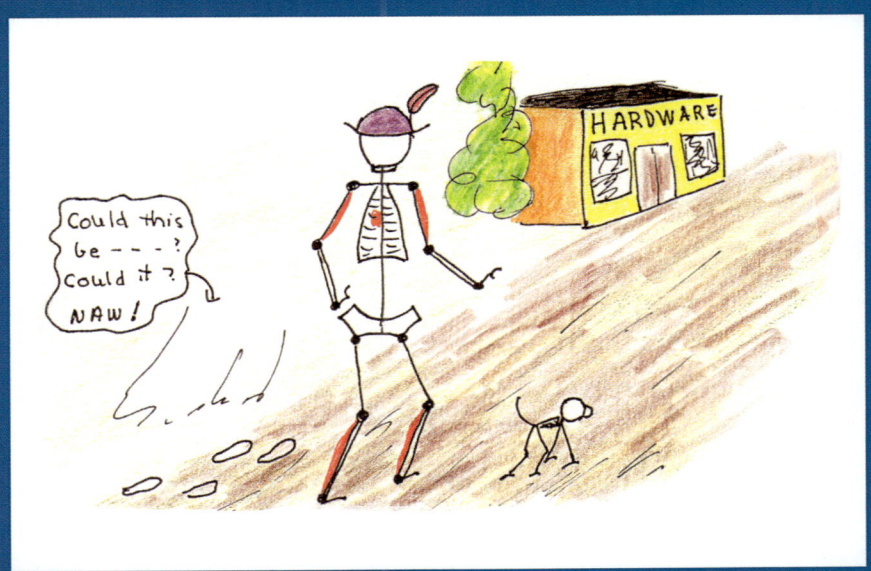

In every house an **ELECTRICAL SYSTEM** is necessary. In our BODY HOUSE the electrical system is the nervous system. It is so critical that the body could not work without it.

Ghost Host and Enod Ton, with Eninac frolicking along beside them, arrived at the hardware store.

Ghost Host was trying explain to Enod Ton about wiring. Enod Ton was not paying attention because he was looking at chicken wire.

"What is this used for, Ghost Host?"

It's chicken wire, Enod Ton. It's used to keep chickens from running all over the yard. You have no use for chicken wire. Eninac, sit still. (Eninac was in the shopping cart, helping with the shopping.) Oh dear! Taking you two shopping is a challenge. Now come over here and let's look at the electrical wire.

Enod Ton looked at Eninac, who was still in the shopping cart wagging his tail. Enod Ton, pushing the cart, loped off after Ghost Host.

As they were walking to the wire department, Ghost Host was explaining why they were talking about wire. We are adding a most important part to your body, Enod Ton. It is called the nervous system, and wire will help me explain. The wiring in a house acts almost like the nerves in the body. Wire carries electrical signals to anything in the house that runs by electricity. The nerves do the same thing for the body. They carry signals to keep your body running.

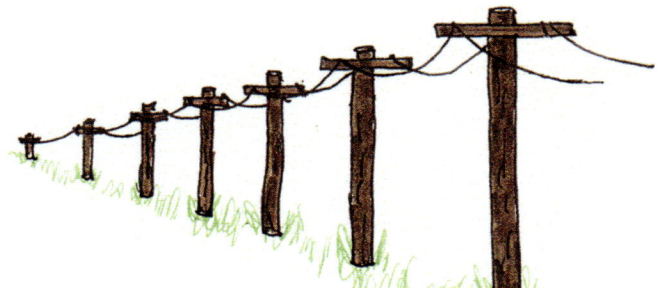

"Well, I am not nervous now. I probably will be after you add it to our 'need-it-now' list. You need this, too, Eninac "said Enod Ton.

Eninac wagged his tail and said" Fra, Fra."

As they reached the wire department, Ghost Host thought about how complicated the whole nervous system is. This is electrical wire, Enod ton. It is covered with a coating to protect the wires. Your nerves are covered with a protective coating, too. When electricity travels over the wires, it goes very fast.

Enod Ton was paying close attention. "This is going to be v-e-r-y interesting, Ghost Host. I understand about the wire and the nerves. Could we go and sit by the lake? I need my books, and Eninac will like watching the ducks."

Excellent Idea, Enod Ton. The little group headed off to the lake for a quiet afternoon of study.

They settled in a comfortable spot where they could enjoy the lake and scenery. Enod Ton had all of his books, falling and scattering as usual. Ghost Host was gathering the books Enod Ton dropped and Eninac's tail was wagging in circles because the lake was a new place.

Now, Enod Ton, look up the nervous system in one of your books.

Enod Ton was flipping pages, saying "hmm" on every page. "Here it is. Look at that! It's everywhere in the body. There are large nerves and tiny ones. The nervous system looks like silver threads."

Yes, it does. Not only that, there are three nervous systems in the body.

Enod Ton fell backward on the grass. "Three! Do you mean that I will have three nervous systems, Ghost Host?"

Right. Let's talk about why there are three nervous systems and what they do.

Enod Ton was recovering from the news that he would have three nervous systems instead of one. He rolled over and crawled through his scattered books. "There must be a book here that tells me why we have three nervous systems. Here's one that says KINDS OF NERVOUS SYSTEMS. Yes. This will be a great help."

HALF TIME

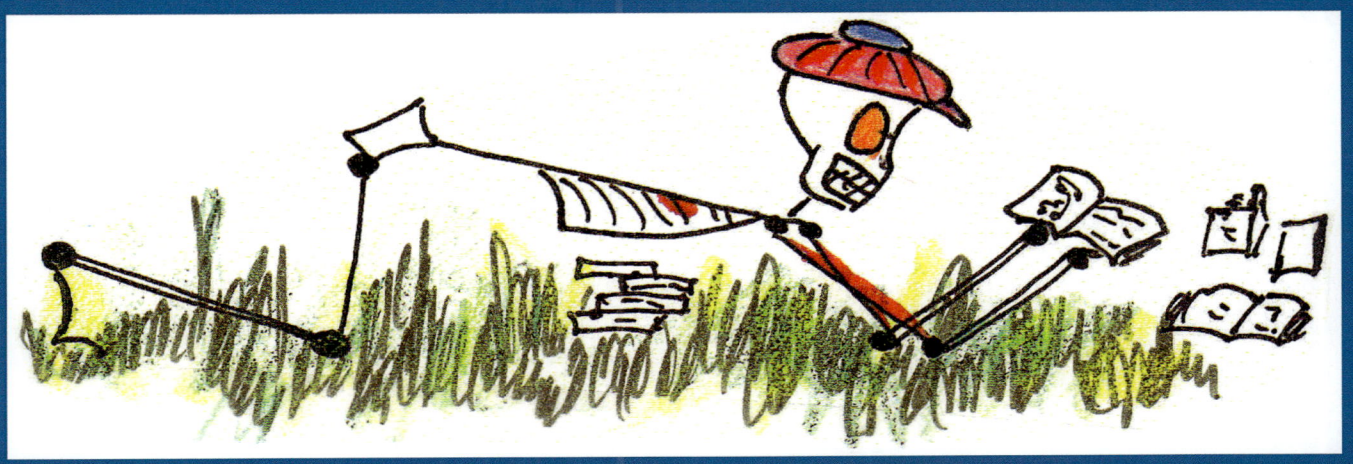

"Hi everyone. This is Enod Ton speaking. What a great job you did with our first five chapters! I think that even Ghost Host is pleased."V

I am more than pleased, Enod Ton. Just look at you. We may have you looking human soon.

"I do seem to have picked up a few body items. I don't think they are particularly pretty but they are necessary. There are still many parts missing. I hope I will get those in the next five chapters."

Ghost Host had a secret surprise for Enod Ton but was determined to keep it a few minutes longer. You don't want to be Enod Ton forever. In five more chapters you will be complete and will have your own "forever" name. Now, Enod Ton, I have a surprise for you.

That got Enod Ton's attention immediately. "What is it? What could it be? Where is it? What is that I hear?"

Enod Ton, I would like you to meet ENINAC. Spell the name backward.

Enod Ton was so pleased that he danced a few steps. "Eninac! How wonderful! I have needed you for a long time. Now we can find parts for both of us."

Eninac was so happy that he barked and wagged his tail at the same time.

"FRA! FRA! " (arf, arf).

Ghost Host smiled a lot.

Off went our happy little group to their next adventure to find the rest of Enod Ton and to find the rest of his friend, Eninac.

ELECTRICAL SYSTEM

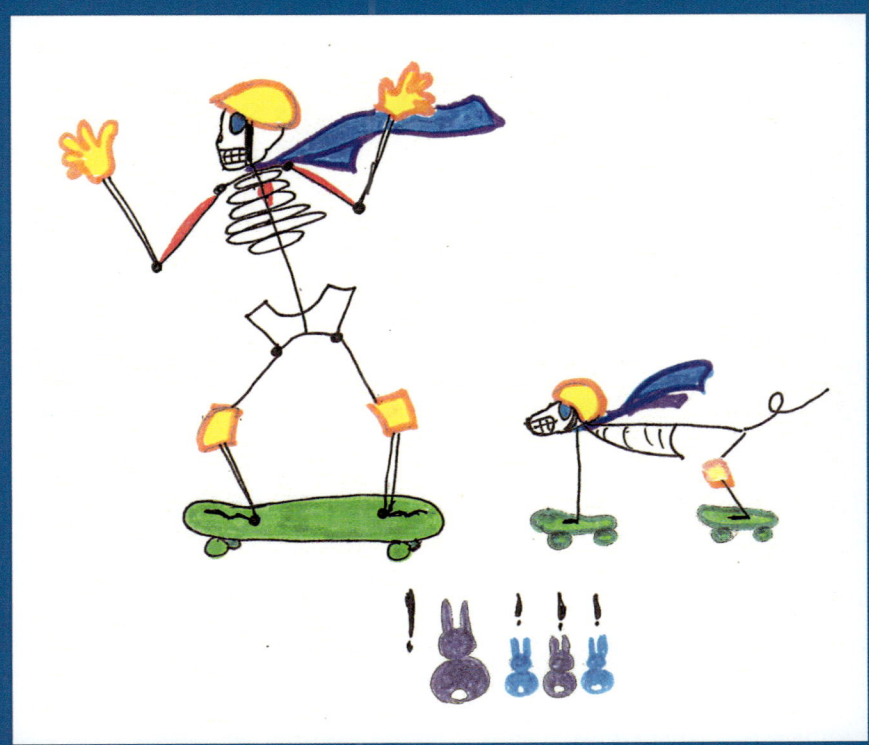

Ghost Host waited for Enod Ton to get settled. Now, first there is the CENTRAL NERVOUS SYSTEM, which is made up of the brain and the spinal cord. It is the most important because everything your body does is directed from these two parts. We will talk much more about the brain in the next chapter. The spinal cord starts in the bottom part of the brain and ends in your lower back. It carries all messages from your brain to the rest of your body. It even sends a few messages by itself. This is the nervous system that tells you to run, walk, carry books and does all of the things you do because you want to.

Enod Ton was still on his knees, looking at his book and listening carefully. "Then my brain will be in my skull and my spinal cord will go down through the holes in my back bone. Oh yes. They are called vertebrae. Here is a picture of that very thing in my book!"

Ghost Host was pleased that Enod Ton remembered the chapter about Framing and where the brain and spinal cord would be placed. Now, the second nervous system is called the AUTONOMIC NERVOUS SYSTEM.

Enod Ton was sitting down and holding several papers. "Wait, Ghost Host. Autonomic sounds like the word automatic. Is that important?"

Yes, it is Enod Ton. The work of the autonomic nervous system is mostly done automatically. This nervous system keeps the internal organs working. Your heart pumps, stomach digests food, lungs take in air and blow it out. All this happens automatically.

Suddenly, Enod Ton understood what Ghost Host was saying. "With this autonomic nervous system, I don't have to think about such things as breathing and digesting food and

heart beat and all of the other things that are working to keep my body going. Ghost Host, I must tell you that I did worry about how this worked. Now I know. I can play soccer and do lots of things and not worry about keeping my heart going.

It is automatic because the autonomic nervous system is doing it for me.

That's Wonderful!"

Ghost Host thought to himself, Enod Ton does understand. Those books and drawings have been a great help. We have the third nervous system, Enod Ton. This one is the most interesting.

Enod Ton snatched a book, flipped rapidly through pages and stopped. "Here it is. Here is the third nervous system. It is called PERIPHERAL NERVOUS SYSTEM. That is a strange name. Why is it called that?"

It is called peripheral because this nervous system works on the parts of your body that are further away from the central nervous system. It is found mostly in the skin.

"Skin! That's right. I will have that, too. So many things! Then, it is this nervous system that tells me when I touch something, or when something touches me."

Ghost Host was so pleased when Enod Ton said that, he jumped up and said HURRAH for you, Enod Ton. What else does it do?

Enod Ton enjoyed Ghost Host's compliment. He thought quickly then said, "If something hurts or if something is hot, the peripheral nervous system tells me, and I move away."

Yes. This nervous system tells you when something is sharp or soft. It tells you if the weather is cold or hot.

"Wait, Ghost Host! I forgot that we need to know about how to dress for the weather. Yes, yes. The peripheral nervous system tells us if the water is too cold for swimming or just right for a shower. Did you hear that Eninac? You had better stay out of the water. It's too cold."

Eninac looked at Enod Ton, then at Ghost Host and said "Fra Fra!"

"Ghost Host, touch my hand so I know where you are. Now close your eyes." Enod Ton had been reading ahead in his NEVER FAIL NERVOUS SYSTEMS book. "I am going to put something in your hand and you tell me what it is." Enod Ton put a ballpoint pen in what he hoped was Ghost Host's hand. "What is it, Ghost Host?"

Ghost Host felt it and said, using my Ghost Power Thinking; it is a ballpoint pen.

"Right, Ghost Host. Now tell me what kind it is and what color."

Ghost Host chuckled. Very funny, Enod Ton. I think that you have been reading the TRICKS TO PLAY ON PEOPLE catalog.

Enod Ton beamed his happiness. "Did you hear that, Eninac? Ghost Host thinks I am getting smarter. I really think so. You are smarter too Eninac."

Eninac wagged his tail. "Fra, Fra"

Ghost Host was proud of Enod Ton because he had learned so much. I have one more question for you, Enod Ton. I identified the pen very quickly. How did that happen?

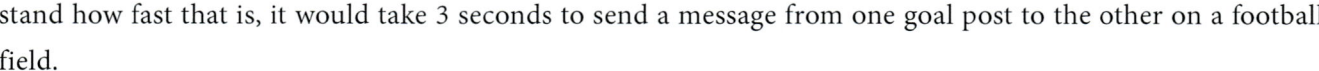

"Very speedy, Ghost Host. Your hand touched the pen and the peripheral nervous system told you what you were touching. I am impressed."

You won't believe this Enod Ton. The average speed a message travels over the nerves is 100 feet per second. Just so you understand how fast that is, it would take 3 seconds to send a message from one goal post to the other on a football field.

Enod Ton rattled to his feet. "Unbelievable, Ghost Host! That is very, very fast." He walked around in a circle, hands in the air. "Learning about the nervous systems has been so complicated. Come Eninac, let's sit down and think about this.

Ghost Host moved over as Enod Ton flopped to the ground and rolled to his back. Eninac rolled over too. You two are a sight. Now, tell me, what was the most important thing you learned?

Enod Ton thought about that for a few seconds. "There are three nervous systems: autonomic, central and peripheral. They all do different jobs but work together. The autonomic nervous system keeps the inside of your body working without you knowing it, like keeping your heart pumping. The central nervous system is the 'boss' of the body. It directs everything the body does like making decisions and sending and receiving messages. The peripheral nervous system sends information from the outer parts of the body to the brain. An example is holding something in your hand with your eyes closed and knowing what it is."

Ghost Host thought to himself that Enod Ton was an excellent student. What is the best thing you have learned, Enod Ton?

"I think the best thing I learned is that I can find thousands of answers in books. I learned that I love to look at books and read about everything."

Ghost Host smiled his secret smile. He looked at Enod Ton and Eninac. They were both napping. He thought he heard a very soft "Fra,Fra."

COMPUTER

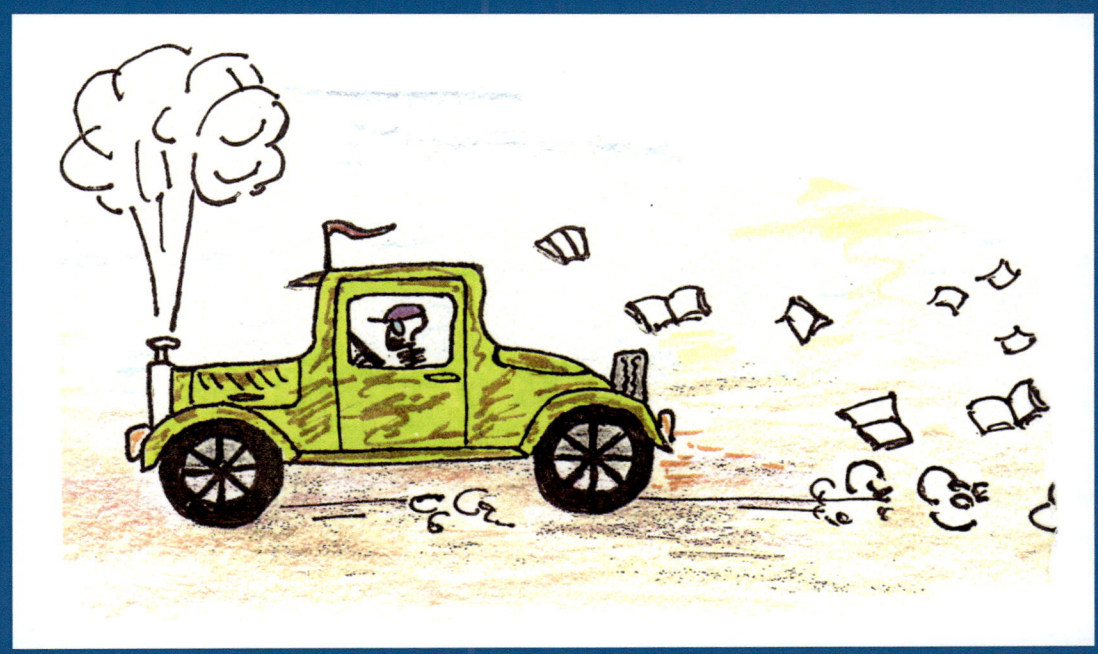

Enod Ton, wake up. It's COMPUTER time. You too, Eninac. This is not the time for sleep. It is the time for learning.

"I am awake, Ghost Host. I can hear you tap dancing on a rock. Eninac, can you hear that? Dancing in the park! Gadzooks! "

Eninac woofed instead of "Fra" (to show that he was bilingual), stretched, yawned and wagged his tail.

Maybe I should sprinkle a little cold water here and there?

"Oh my! Jump up and smile Eninac We are awake, Ghost Host. Look at Eninac. He is smiling. So am I. Did I hear you say computer?"

Eninac was still smiling. He managed a woof.

You did, Enod Ton and we are about to begin our study of the brain, which is the computer of the body. It controls absolutely everything.

"I hope that it soon controls your dancing Ghost Host. What was that noisy dance step, you were doing?"

What nonsense, Enod ton. You had better gather up your books and papers. It looks like rain. We will go to my house to study and have tea and cookies.

"That is an excellent idea, Ghost Host. Help me with this, Eninac. I know that Ghost Host will be in a hurry because cookies are involved." Eninac scratched a few papers and picked up a book in his mouth. Enod Ton had his arms full of books. They scurried off after Ghost Host.

When everyone was settled in Ghost Host's living room and the tea and cookies were ready, they went to work.

Enod Ton was trying to get all of his books in order. "There, I think everything is ready. I have many books about the brain." Enod Ton opened several of them, all with pictures and drawings of the brain. "I don't think that it looks like a computer."

Of course it doesn't look like a computer, Enod Ton. It looks like a brain. We call it the body's computer because it controls everything the body does. It is also the thinking department.

"Let me think, Ghost Host. Wait a minute. What did I just say? Let me

Think--?' I have been thinking all along. Answering questions is thinking. Right?"

Right! We are on track, Enod Ton. Have some tea and give Eninac a cookie.

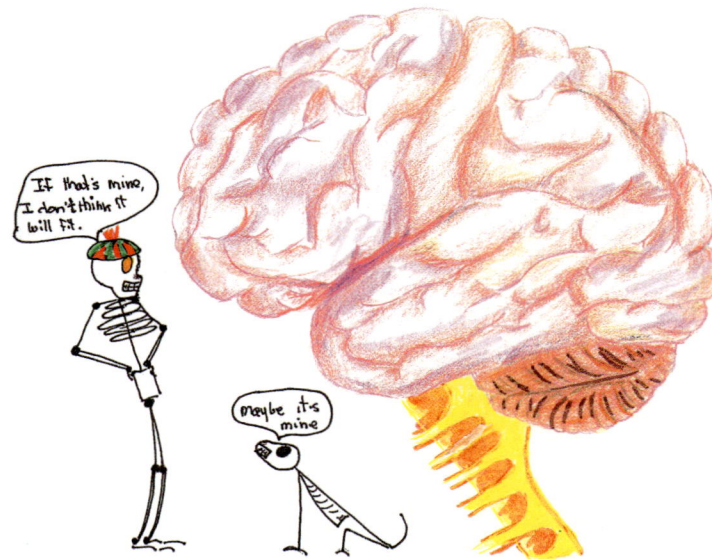

Enod Ton studied the pictures of the brain. "So that's what a brain looks like. It looks very complicated."

Oh, it is very complicated, Enod Ton. We are going to study only a very small part of what it does. If you decide to become a brain surgeon, you can study the rest of it.

"Hmmm, brain surgeon. I'll have to think about that. Ghost Host, if I look at the brain from the front, it looks like there are two brains. Can that be?"

Yes, there are actually two brains. They are called the right brain and the left-brain.

The right side of the brain controls the left side of the body. Think about that. The left-brain controls the right side of the body

"Whoa, Ghost Host. Do you mean that I will have two separate brains?

How do the two work together? "

The two sides of the brain are connected but you can't see the connection. They do work together very well. The two large parts you are looking at are called cerebral hemispheres, or cerebrum for short.

"Cerebrum, yes. The book says the cerebrum is divided into work areas. Each area does a different job. Let me draw a picture of the brain and show you where the areas are and what they do."

Ghost Host was eating cookies and drinking tea. Eninac was eating cookies. That is wonderful, Enod Ton. With that drawing, our student guests can understand the different parts of the brain.

Enod Ton was so busy looking at the areas of the cerebrum; he forgot to have his cookies. "This part of the brain has a memory storage place. It is a little like a built-in library. The book shows other parts of the brain. Could we talk about those?"

You are so good at those drawings, Enod Ton. Would you do another drawing showing all of the brain? Then we will explain the parts.

Enod Ton jumped to his feet with crayons in hand and set about drawing a large picture of the brain and all of its departments. As he was drawing, Enod Ton said "I read about these parts and I would like to be the teacher this time."

A fine idea, Enod Ton. I shall have another cup of tea and Eninac and I shall have

A few more cookies and listen.

Enod Ton thought to himself, "Hmm --a few more cookies? More like a few dozen."

Enod Ton set about drawing the other parts of the brain. He hummed to himself as he worked.

Ghost Host was watching Enod Ton. What is that you are singing?

"It was 'You Go To My Head', I think. What do you think it was?"

I'm not sure Enod Ton. It could have been "Lost In Space".

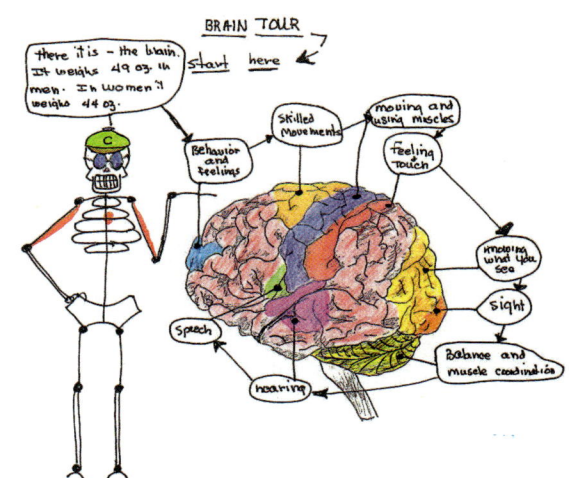

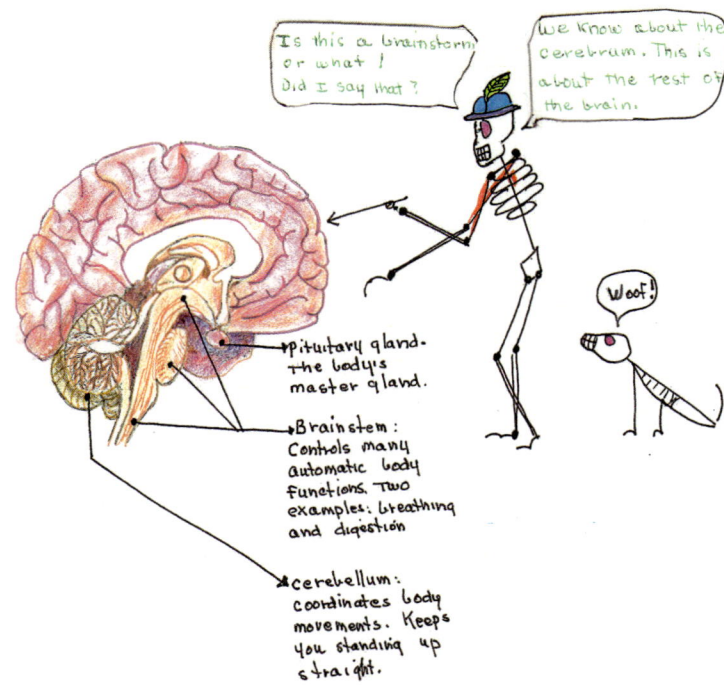

Enod Ton made a great show of sighing, and finished the drawing. "There, now. If you will follow the drawing from the top, it will explain everything. Our bodies will not work without the parts of the brain I have drawn. Eninac, pay attention. You will have a brain, too."

Eninac wagged his tail and said "fra, fra, -- woof." He was being bilingual again.

Ghost Host was listening to both Enod Ton and Eninac. Why don't you look up what a dog's brain looks like? Eninac would like to see that.

Eninac wagged his tail in a circle and said "woof, woof, woooof."

Enod Ton looked at Eninac and said, "Of course you would like to see your brain. I shall look for it immediately." Enod Ton set about flipping pages and papers, littering the floor with notes and pencils. "Get ready, Eninac. I found it!"

Ghost Host, Enod Ton and Eninac looked at the dog's brain. "Look at that!" said Enod Ton.

Eninac looked at the picture, ran around in a small circle and said "Woof, Woof".

Everyone was surprised at the different kinds of brains. Ghost Host said Look at the drawing of the frog's brain. It is small and not too complicated. A frog does not need a large, complicated brain to hop about and say "RIBIT – RIBIT". Now look at the drawing of the dog's brain. It is different because a dog lives a more complicated life and he needs more "brain power".

Enod Ton looked at Eninac. "I can see that you are a very smart dog, Eninac. Smart dogs help clean up the floor" Eninac sat down. He was probably thinking that was "people work".

Ghost Host and Enod Ton sat down on the floor. There were books, papers, pencils, crayons and cookie crumbs scattered everywhere. Just think about what we have learned, Enod Ton. The brain controls everything.

Enod Ton was thinking about all of the brain. "Yes, everything. The brain even has areas to store what we have learned. I feel like my storage area is full, Ghost Host. Could we learn about that tomorrow?"

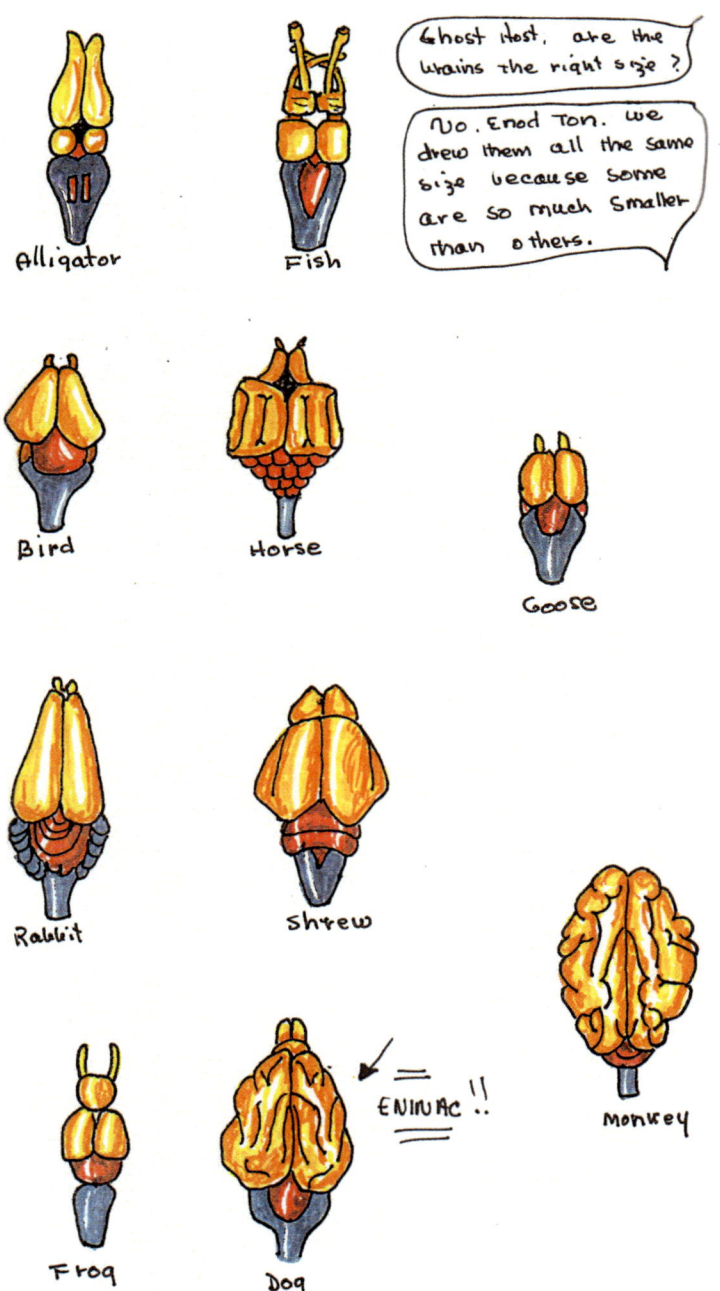

Ghost Host looked around the living room. Brains can sleep only after they help clean up living rooms, Enod Ton.

"You are fooling me, Ghost Host. I will help clean up because I made most of the mess. Look what I found! It says 'Sensors'. It looks so interesting."

That is what we will study next, Enod Ton. Right now we should go to bed.

Enod Ton agreed with that. "Where is Eninac?"

There was a sleepy "woof" from the corner of the couch.

SENSORS

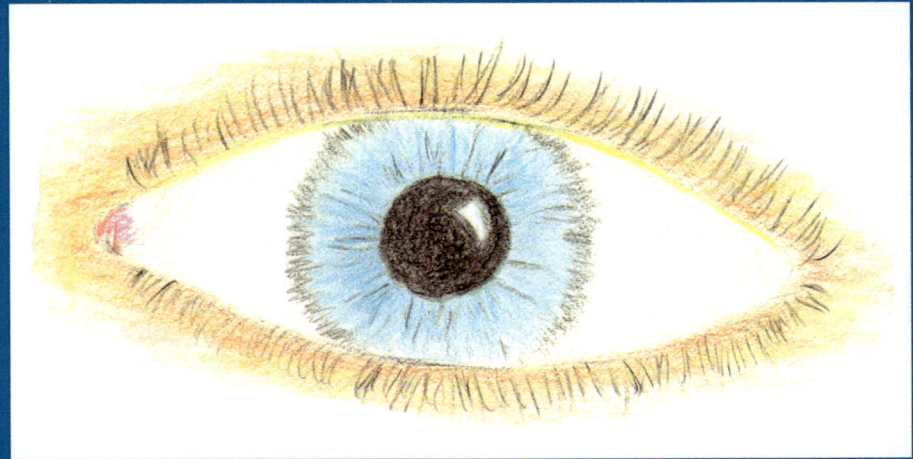

Houses have a system of **SENSORS**. A few examples of house sensors are the thermostat for heating and cooling the house, motion lights and smoke alarms.

Ghost Host was having cereal. Eninac was looking out the window, watching the birds. Enod Ton was sitting on the floor in the middle of his books, flipping pages.

This is good cereal, Enod Ton. Have some.

"Ummm. It is good. Look at the bubbles, and I can hear them pop!"

Right, Enod Ton! You have just found our five senses.

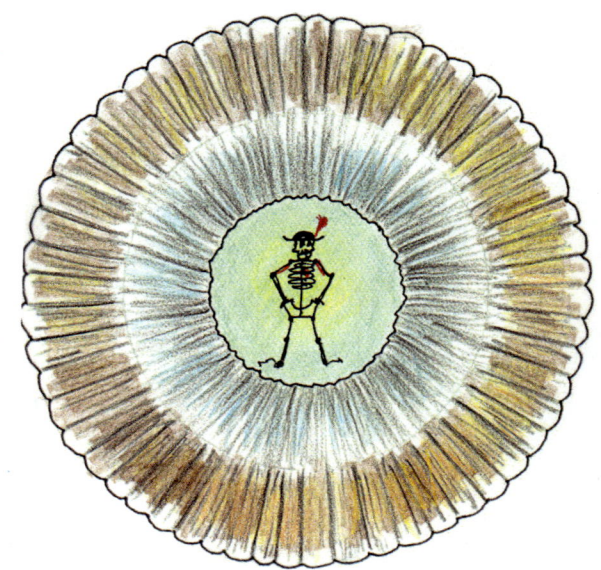

Enod Ton was very surprised. "I did that? How did that happen?"

Ghost Host settled into a comfortable chair. Let me answer your question with a question. Look at your books, Enod Ton. How many senses do we have?

Enod Ton found the right book and looked at the Table of Contents. "Here it is! Senses Of The Body. There are five main senses."

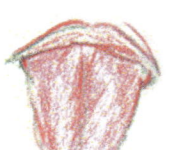

A moment ago you were surprised that you gave us clues to the five senses. Let's name them.

"Yes, let me. There are SIGHT, HEARING, TOUCH, TASTE and SMELL."

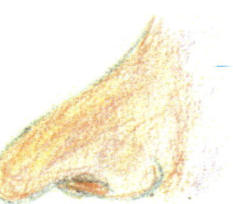

Enod Ton was pleased with his discovery. He was so interested in what he had found that he scrabbled about in a few more books.

Ghost Host had drawings of where the senses are located. Look at this, Enod Ton.

Here are examples of where we find them.

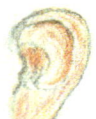 Enod Ton looked closely at the drawings. "Let's go back to the cereal, Ghost Host. I could see it, hear it pop, feel it in my mouth, taste it and smell it. That's how I found the five senses."

Exactly, Enod Ton. Each sense is amazing. Let's look at them separately.

"Oh good! I would like that. Eninac, stop watching the birds and come sit with me on the floor. I believe there is a milk bone for you."

Eninac came quickly. The milk bone helped.

Ghost Host had placed several large charts on the wall. I think that we should start with the eye, Enod Ton. We use our sight most of all. As you can see - ha - use your eyes, Enod Ton. The eye is round and mostly white.

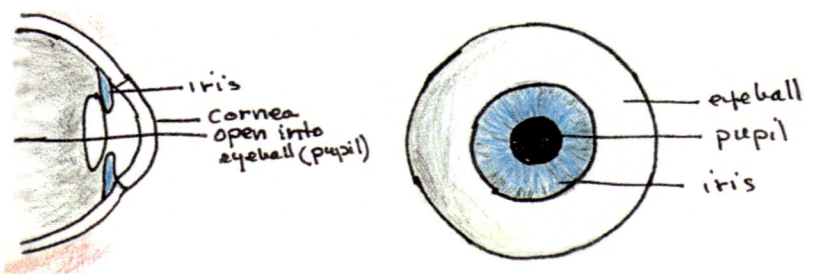

"But Ghost Host, people's eyes are brown or blue or green or other colors. You said eyes are mostly white."

Look at the chart, Enod Ton. The eye is like a ball and the outside of it is white. There is color, but only on the front. What other color do you see?

Enod Ton looked closely at the chart. "I see black, too."

What you are seeing is not a color. It is a hole called the pupil. You are looking right into the eyeball.

"Into the eyeball? Let me look at your eyes, Ghost Host. Wait a minute. Do ghosts have eyes? "

Of course ghosts have eyes! I may even have radar, you never know.

"I knew that! Ghosts are supposed to have 'eye holes'. Could you make your eye appear so that I can look? Your eyes are brown.

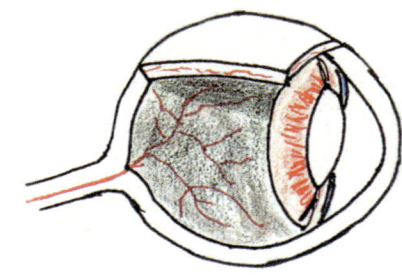

51

My oh my! Ghost Host, I just thought of something. If you are a ghost, how can I see your eye?"

Because I let you see it, Silly. Real ghosts can appear or totally disappear if they want to. It is our special Ghost Energy.

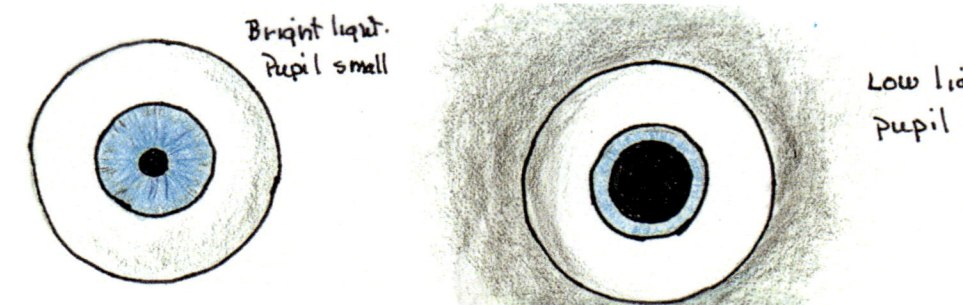

"Oooooooh. I am impressed!"

Now Enod Ton, remember, the eyeball is white. There is one spot on the eyeball that is not white. Look at the chart. There is a clear spot and that is what you see through. It is called the cornea.

Enod Ton peered closely at the chart. "Yes, I see it. The colored part of your eye is right behind the cornea."

That colored part of your eye is the iris. Right in the middle of the iris is the pupil. Remember, that is the hole that goes into your eye.

"Yes, I remember. Ghost Host, sometimes the pupil is tiny and sometimes it is large. Why does this happen?"

Ghost Host was happy with Enod Ton's question. The inside of your eye is very sensitive. The pupil controls the amount of light going into your eye. If you are out in the sun, the pupil gets very small to keep out too much light. If you are in a dark room, the pupil gets large because it opens to let in more light.

"That is a miracle! And Ghost Host, I know how that happens!"

Ghost Host stopped flipping charts. Tell us how that happens, Enod Ton.

Enod Ton jumped to his feet, papers flying in all directions. Even Eninac wagged his tail. "The pupil gets larger and smaller automatically. This is done by the autonomic nervous system! How wonderful. I thought of that!"

Ghost Host did a small dance step. YES! You are getting very good at this!

Enod Ton glowed with praise. He picked up Eninac, scratched where his ear would be and sat down.

Ghost Host remembered another thing about eyes. We had better talk a bit about "seeing", Enod Ton. Do you know how we see?

Enod Ton thought for a moment. "Uh, well, not exactly. You are the only one who can explain things when they are complicated, Ghost Host."

Thank you for the compliment, Enod Ton. Now -- how do we see? People and many animals have eyes that are made to see well in light and not so well in the dark. Some animals, like cats, see well in both dark and light. When we look at something, like a ball, the light reflects off the ball and into our eyes. That reflection hits the inside of the eye. A message goes to the brain that the eye is seeing something. The brain sorts out what it is, and you know that you are seeing a ball.

Enod ton sat up and listened closely. "Then the brain can even tell us what kind of ball it is, and what it is used for. Now I know how it works!" It's AUTOMATIC!"

Now, Enod Ton, how do you know what I have been telling you?

"Because I heard what you were saying – uh, oh! I know what you are going to say. You are going to ask HOW I knew what you are saying. That is our sense of hearing."

Hoho, Enod Ton. You are getting smarter every hour. Would you like to explain how we hear?

"Yes! That would be great fun."

Enod Ton leaped to his feet, took the pointer and zipped through the drawings until he came to the drawing of the ear.

"Are you ready, Ghost Host? And Eninac, you listen, too. Dogs have very sharp hearing."

Ghost Host had some toast with peanut butter and jelly. Eninac had a milk bone. They were ready to listen.

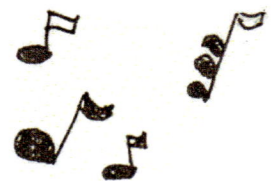

"We are going to take a trip into your ear. First, I must tell you the ear has three parts: the external ear, middle ear and inner ear. The part we see is on the outside with folds is part of the external ear and is called the PINNA. The folds are there to catch all kinds of sounds. Now its experiment time. With the tip of your finger, push the outside of the pinna against your head. What does it do to your hearing? Right! You do not hear as well because the pinna is not catching as many sounds."

Enod Ton took a deep breath and continued. "Now, put your finger behind your pinna and push it forward. What happens? Sounds are louder because your pinna is catching more sound."

Ghost Host nodded happily and Eninac said "Fra, Fra".

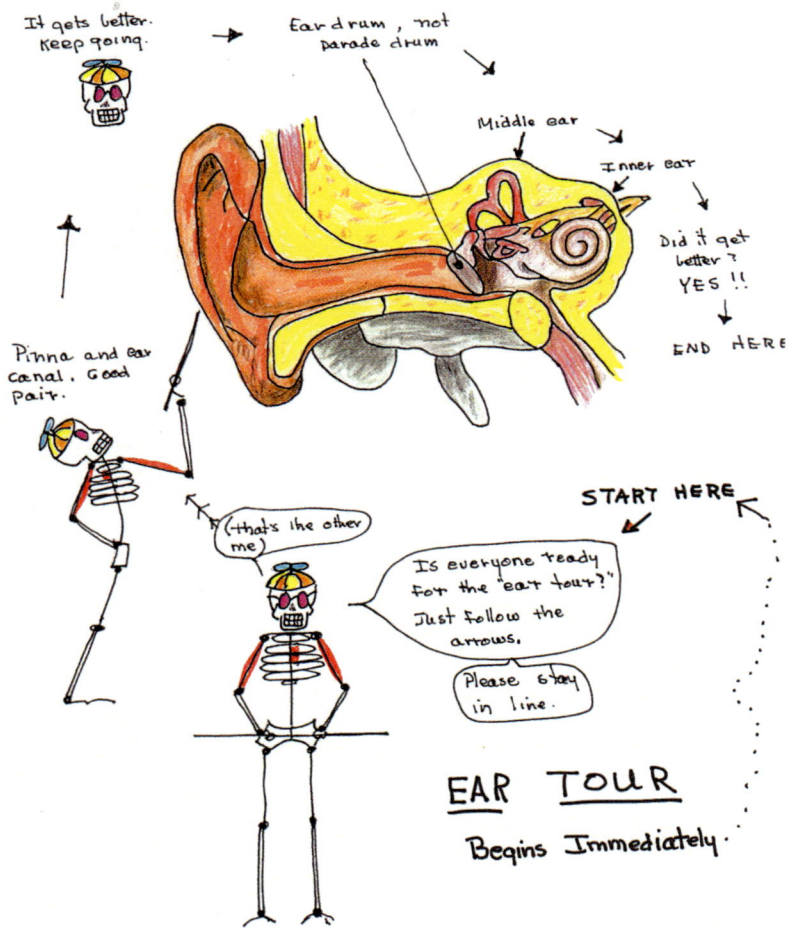

Enod Ton was ready to continue. "The other part of the external ear is a tube called EAR CANAL. It ends at the EAR DRUM. The ear canal is like a tunnel. It carries sound to the ear drum."

Ghost Host wanted to make sure that everyone understood about the eardrum. Enod Ton, think about a parade. In the marching bands there are always drums. When the drum is hit with the drumstick it makes a booming sound because the drum vibrates. Your eardrum is a little like a parade drum. Instead of a drumstick hitting your ear drum, sound hits it and makes it vibrate.

"I was coming to that, Ghost Host, but you explained it better. When sound hits the eardrum, the vibrations go from the eardrum, through the middle ear, into the inner ear and a message is sent to the brain. The brain identifies the sound, and you know what you are hearing."

Ghost Host was humming and pretending to ignore Enod Ton.

"I know what that tune is, Ghost Host! It is 'Yankee Doodle'. Does that mean it is the 4th of July?"

Ghost Host laughed and said Of course it is not the 4th of July. How did you know I was humming 'Yankee Doodle'?

Enod Ton stopped what he was doing. "My ears caught the sound and my brain identified it. You are tricky, Ghost Host."

You are a miracle, Enod Ton. Now, close your eyes and put out your hand. Ghost Host put an ice cube into Enod Ton's hand. What is that?

"It is an ice cube."

How do you know it is an ice cube?

"Because I can feel it. Uh-oh, you fooled me again, Ghost Host. I know what you are going to say. This is the third sense -TOUCH."

Right. Let me ask you a question, Enod Ton. How does a person walk?

Enod Ton stood up and walked about. "A person puts one foot on the floor, then the other."

How do you know that your feet are on the floor?

"You can feel the floor. You did it again, Ghost Host! You fooled me! That is our sense of touch."

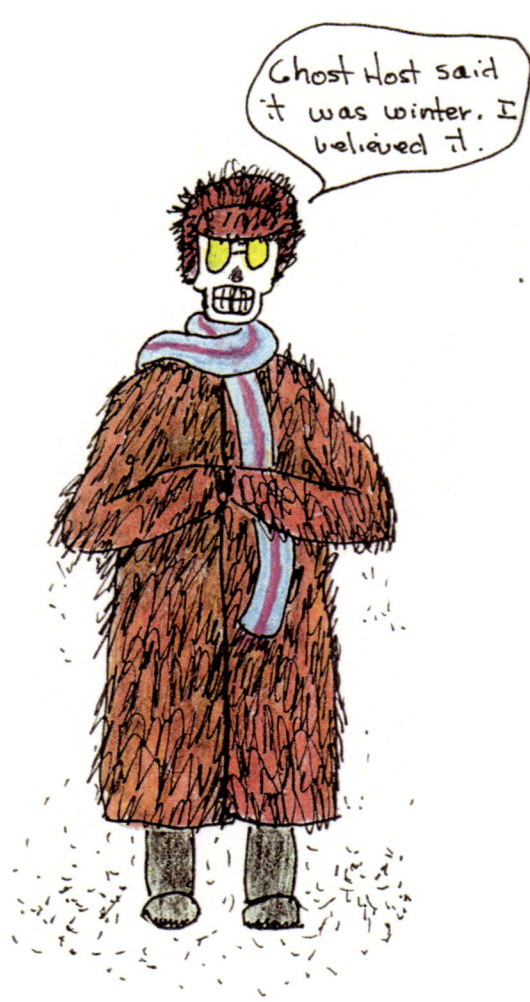

Our whole body is covered with the sensation of touch. There are some places that are more sensitive to touch than others. Let me name a few: hands, feet, nose, face, and neck.

Enod Ton was turning the pages of one of his books very fast. "I found it! Something else our sense of touch does. It tells us if the weather is hot or cold.

That means our sense of touch tells us what kind of clothes to wear."

Our sense of touch does many more things, but there is one we should mention. Touch warns us about painful things. If someone steps on your toe, it hurts. The sense of touch tells us what is painful and we stay away from what will hurt us.

"Well Ghost Host, we have a built-in warning system. One more thing that is a 'body miracle'. I made that up. Grand, isn't it?"

Enod Ton was so pleased with himself that he went to the cookie jar and had four cookies. He gave one to Eninac. "These are good cookies, Ghost Host. I especially like the ones with nuts in them. Would you like one?"

Ghost Host took a cookie. You are right, Enod Ton, they are outstanding cookies.

"Ah-Ah, Ghost Host! How do you know they are that good? I think I fooled YOU this time!"

You did! I know the cookies are good because of our senses of taste and smell. These two work together. We have already talked about the taste buds on the tongue.

"Yes, there are four different kinds of taste buds on the tongue; sweet, sour, salt and bitter."

True. Smell and taste are connected. You can't taste anything if your sense of smell is not working.

"Why would smell not be working?"

If you hold your nose and eat something, you can't taste it. If you have a bad cold and your nose is stopped up, you can't taste.

"HO! I shall make a vow never to catch a cold because I want to taste everything!'"

Well, good luck, Enod Ton. That cold may catch you! Before you think about that, there is something that we should look at a little more closely. We have already said that taste will not work without smell.

"I know. Clogged noses and such. Here is a question for you, Ghost Host. Does the sense of smell work without the sense of taste?"

Enod Ton, you are ahead of me. That is what we want to look at more closely. Yes, the sense of smell will work without the taste sense. Eninac will have a better sense of smell than we do.

"Did you hear that, Eninac? You smell better than we do. Uh -oh. I think that's wrong. Let me say that again. It means that people don't smell so good. There still seems to be something wrong with that, too. Oh Dear! I am in a word mess."

Ghost Host was laughing. Eninac said "Woof. Fra. Fra. Woof." Enod Ton was still muttering about who did not smell good.

Ghost Host was trying to stop laughing. It's time we think about all that we have found out about the senses. To do that quickly, let's consider a carrot. We SEE it and know it is a carrot. We can even HEAR it crunching when we take a bite. We can FEEL it crunching. Take another bite. It TASTES like a carrot. Sniff. What does it SMELL like? A carrot. IT MUST BE A CARROT! We have used all five of our senses to know that it is, indeed a carrot.

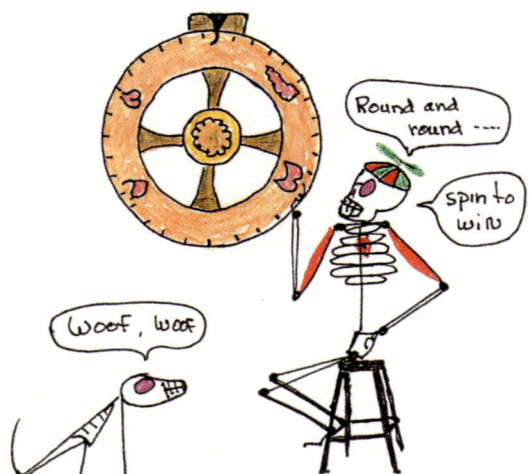

Enod Ton had not quite recovered from the smell experience but he was trying. "I will think about that for a while, Ghost Host. Right now I need a rest."

DUCTWORKS

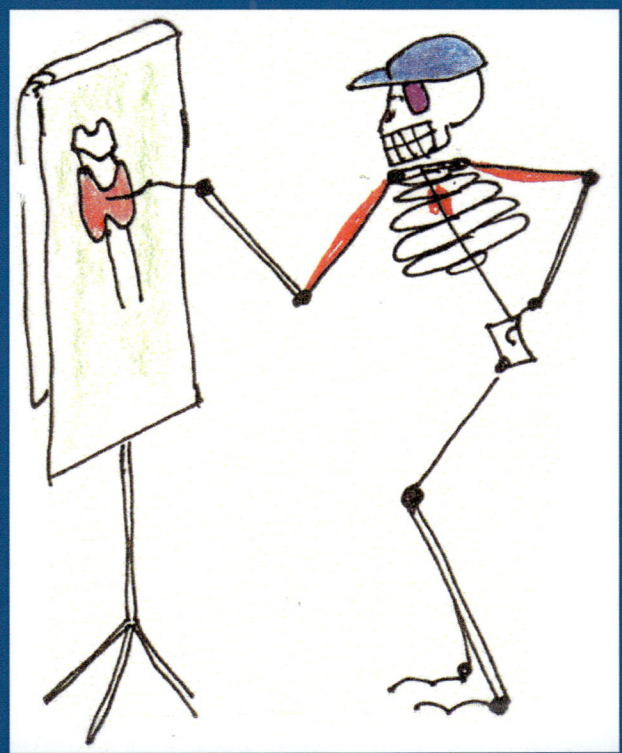

Enod Ton, the DUCTWORKS are another part for your BODY HOUSE. Houses sometimes need to be made larger because people need more space. Bodies are much the same. They need more space too, so they can grow.

"Another part! I am being stuffed! I won't ask where this is to go. You will tell me that it will all fit.

And you will tell me that I cannot live without whatever it is. Well, I don't know."

You are such a worrywart, Enod Ton. You hit it right when you said everything would fit and that you cannot live without it - or I should say "them".

"THEM! Oh Dear."

Ha. Yes. Many. "M-A-N-Y?"

I cannot keep you in suspense any longer, Enod Ton. I am talking about glands. There are so many glands in the body that I am going to leave most of them as a surprise so that you can discover them for yourself. You love to read and I know that you will look all of them up in your great supply of books.

"Do I need a rest before we start?"

No, but an apple may help. Please munch quietly. Eninac, have a milk bone.

Since Eninac liked milk bones, he said "Woof, woof."

Two of the glands we will talk about have to do with our bodies expanding and growing. They are the PITUITARY and the THYROID. We will also need to know about the ADRENAL and PARATHYROID glands.

"Wait, Ghost Host. You know that I have to see drawings of these things." Enod Ton scurried after his books. He flipped through many pages, and found the section titled GLANDS. "Here's the pituitary gland. Let's start with it."

Good choice. It is what we call the Master Gland. It is the size of a small peanut and you can see that it is well hidden under the brain. I like to call it "The Boss".

"That sounds like it is a powerful gland. I think I should have a lot of respect for the pituitary gland. What does it do, Ghost Host?"

The pituitary has many jobs to do. The one you will be most interested in is growing. It has coded information to tell your body when to grow. It sends messages to other growth glands to begin body expansion. Since this is the boss, the other glands get to work.

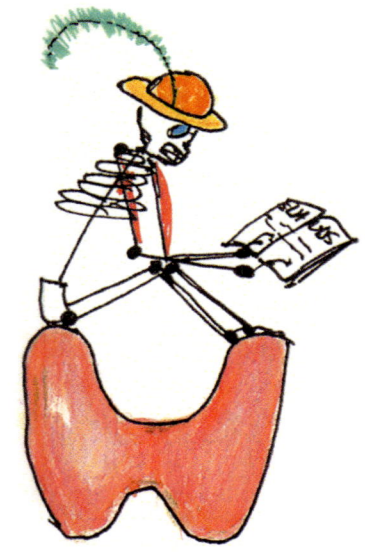

"Now I understand why small children 'grow up'". Enod Ton smiled secretly. "Why, Ghost Host, are you sure that children don't grow down?"

Very funny, Enod Ton. You probably have a "funny" gland. Now tell me, does the pituitary gland work all of the time, or just when a person is growing?

Enod Ton looked through his <u>Handy Guide To Glands</u> book. " It is always working. Whether you are running about playing an exciting game or you are sitting down to dinner, your body adjusts to whatever you are doing. The pituitary helps with this. If you have a cold or the flu, your body must adjust to that on the inside. The pituitary gland helps with all of this."

Enod Ton, you are a fountain of knowledge. I am most impressed.

"This little, peanut size gland does all of this? I am still reading my trusty books. I shall be respectful and kind to the pituitary. Do you think that will help, Ghost Host?"

By all means, Enod Ton. You might also try eating right, getting enough rest and exercise.

"I shall practice resting right now, Ghost Host."

Good. While you are resting, we will go on to the next gland. It is called the THYROID. It is located in your throat right under your larynx. Remember the larynx from our study of VENTILATION?

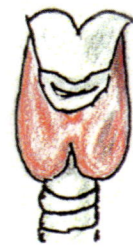

"Yes, I do. It is the larynx or voice box. It is one of my favorite parts of the body."

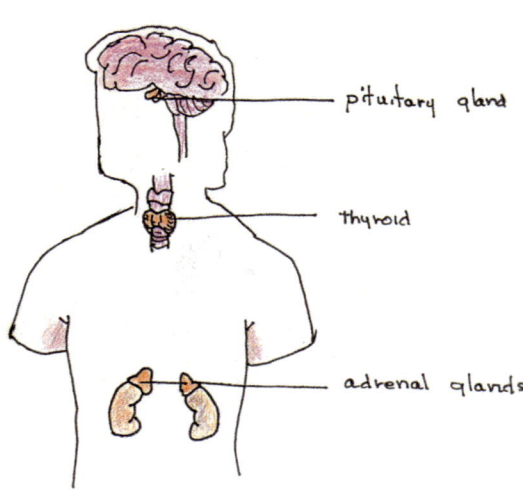

How well I know that! The thyroid has a lot to do with body weight and how we grow. It also produces small amounts of iodine.

"IODINE! You mean that I will have iodine inside my body? You mean that my insides will be the color of iodine? Iodine stings. I don't want iodine -- do I?" Enod Ton had jumped to his feet to look at the drawing.

Ghost Host was sitting down laughing at Enod Ton. Honestly, Enod Ton. Nothing will be thecolor of iodine. It will not sting. It is one of the necessary parts of your body chemistry. Ghost Host was still laughing but Enod Ton could not see this.

"W-E-L-L, that's a relief. Whew! "

Now Enod Ton, you were excited and jumping about just then. At that moment, you were using another gland and you did not know it.

"Am I up to hearing about this? I feel weak from something."

Oh, I think that you can. When you got excited, your ADRENAL gland went to work and gave you an extra energy boost.

"Adrenal gland? Another one! Just a moment. I have my handy gland book. Adrenal, adrenal. Ah, here it is. Look at that! It looks like a little clown hat. What is it sitting on?"

It is sitting on a kidney, Enod Ton. That is where it lives.

"Well, that is much better looking than the thyroid gland with its iodine."

I do hope that you stop worrying about that iodine. Let's think about the adrenal glands. One of the things these glands do is make a chemical called adrenaline. In an emergency, the adrenaline gives you extra energy and strength.

"That is a grand plan, Ghost Host. We all meet emergencies once in a while. What would be an example of one?"

You are riding your bicycle and a car backs out of a driveway in front of you. You put on your brakes so fast that you may not remember doing it. When you stop, you feel a bit weak from the scare, and from the extra adrenaline the glands have given you. The adrenaline helped you stop in a hurry.

"I understand that. If we get excited about something, we have extra adrenaline working, too. If I won a new bicycle, I would certainly use a lot of adrenaline."

Of course you would. If Eninac saw or heard something strange, he would get excited and bark. He would be using his adrenaline. That is his way of telling us that there is something we should know.

"I can see that the adrenal glands are an important addition to the BODY HOUSE. I have to think about the glands we have talked about. The pituitary is the master gland and controls the other glands. The thyroid helps control growth and weight (and has iodine) - sigh!"

Get on with it, Enod Ton. Remember your adrenaline.

"Ah yes. Those I like - the adrenal glands. They are going to help me win a bicycle."

I see I have another problem. They won't help you WIN a bicycle, Enod Ton. They will help you celebrate IF you win.

"Drat! I thought I had you fooled, Ghost Host. I would rather ride in your funny car. It holds all of my books and cookies and Eninac."

Why do I worry about you, Enod Ton? I should know by now that you are a great "fooler". You mentioned all of your books. Your assignment is to read about all of the other glands. That should keep you busy for days. Well, maybe hours.

"I need a slight rest to get my adrenaline ready. Let's go get an ice cream and give Eninac a milk bone."

They all hurried to Ghost Host's funny car and off they went in a cloud of rust.

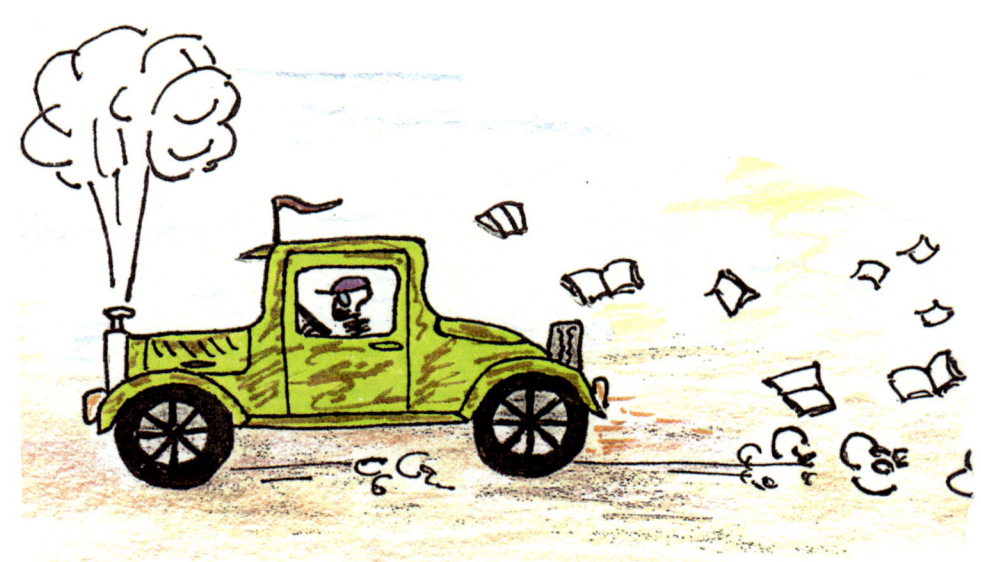

WATERPROOFING AND PROTECTION

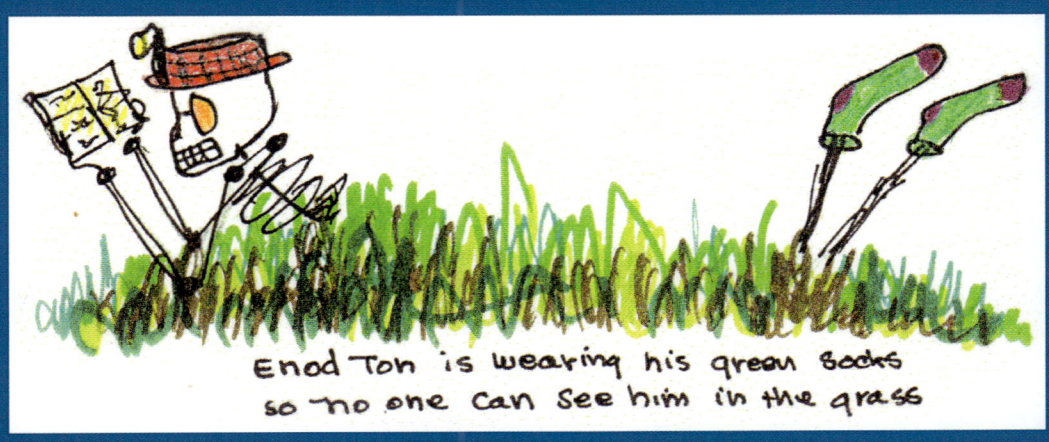

Enod Ton is wearing his green socks so no one can see him in the grass

Now we have to do some **WATERPROOFING** and **PROTECTION** for all of the organs and parts we have put together to make you, Enod Ton, a person, and you, Eninac, a fully equipped dog.

Enod Ton and Ghost Host were all resting in the park. Eninac was frolicking by the lake, watching the ducks.

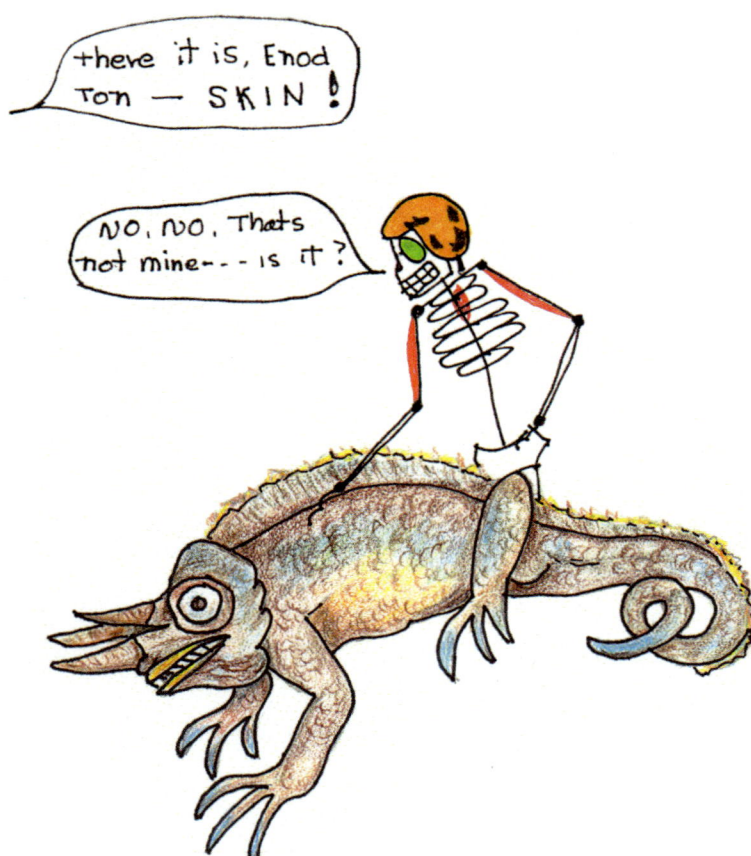

What a nice breeze this afternoon, Ghost Host remarked.

Enod Ton said, "I don't feel any breeze."

Of course you don't. There is another part of the BODY HOUSE, which you need to feel most anything. Prepare yourself Enod Ton. This is the largest organ of the WHOLE body.

Enod Ton fell backward on the grass. "Even my adrenalin won't save me from this shock. The biggest organ? There is simply no room for ANYTHING else in my body. How big is it? No, don't tell me. No matter what you say, it is too much. Would it fit in a backpack?"

A backpack! You ARE in shock. Who said that it was for IN your body? Guess again, Enod Ton.

"Not IN my body. Hmmm. Wait a minute. I KNOW WHAT IT IS! I KNOW! It is SKIN!"

The very thing. The skin is the first thing the world sees when they meet you. I might even say you have it all over you.

"All over me. Ghost Host, I am trying to think that was funny. Now I must think seriously about this. I never thought of the skin as an organ - like the stomach, or something."

Well, now you have a new way of thinking about the skin. You can't leave home without it and besides; you are going to like what you hear. The skin does so many things.

"So many? I thought that it only covered the entire outside of the body. What else does it do?"

Your books are in the car. Run and get them and we will explore all of the wonders of the skin.

Enod Ton raced off across the grass with Eninac after him, woofing and wagging his tail.

Enod Ton returned with his arms full of books, dropping all sorts of papers. Eninac was following, halfheartedly chasing the papers. He really had his eye on the ducks.

If we explore and study anything else, I will have to trade in my beautiful little car for a truck with a shell over the truck bed or a bookmobile.

"Oh no, Ghost Host. I like your car. I even like the rust. Why would you trade it away?"

Because of your traveling library, Enod Ton.

Enod Ton was secretly laughing. He knew Ghost Host would not trade his rusty little car for anything.

You asked what else the skin does besides cover your body. First of all, it is waterproof. It is better than any raincoat. It protects your body from sunrays, injury and infection.

"Well, think of that! I would like to add one more thing. The skin also helps to hold us together like a big sack."

That is another way of looking at it, Enod Ton. It does help the muscles keep everything under control. There are several other things I know you would be interested in.

"I have my books all ready and have found 'skin' in four of them. Well look at that. I did not realize that skin had layers. "

Each of the layers has a purpose. If we talked about all of them, we would be here for a week. We will talk about two. Let's start with the top layer, which we see when we look at someone. Then we can talk about the lower layer. The top layer has folds, and cracks, and tiny holes and ---

"Wait a minute Ghost Host. HOLES? Won't water and dirt get in? I don't want holes in my skin."

Oh Dear! Another trauma. You will have them anyway, Enod Ton. They are pores and they keep your body air-conditioned. Let me explain how they work.

"Good. What do you mean 'air conditioned'?"

When the weather is hot, the pores open and send a watery material to the surface of the skin. This is called PERSPIRATION or SWEAT. As it dries, it cools your skin.

"Yes, yes! What about when I get cold?"

Your skin takes care of that, too.

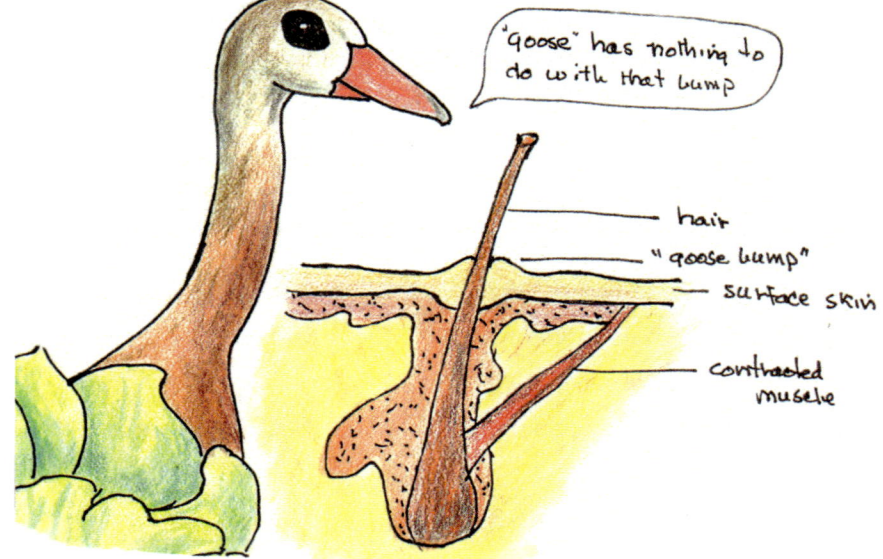

When you get cold or are afraid of something, your skin responds and closes the pores automatically. The little muscles at the bottom of the skin hair make the hair stand up. That is what makes "goose bumps". All of this keeps your body heat inside.

"GOOSE BUMPS! That makes me want to sit down and have a cookie and think about it. Cookies help me think clearly."

Help you think clearly? Enod Ton, you will use any excuse to have a cookie. If your thinking has cleared up, Let's get along with our skin discussion. There is a lot more.

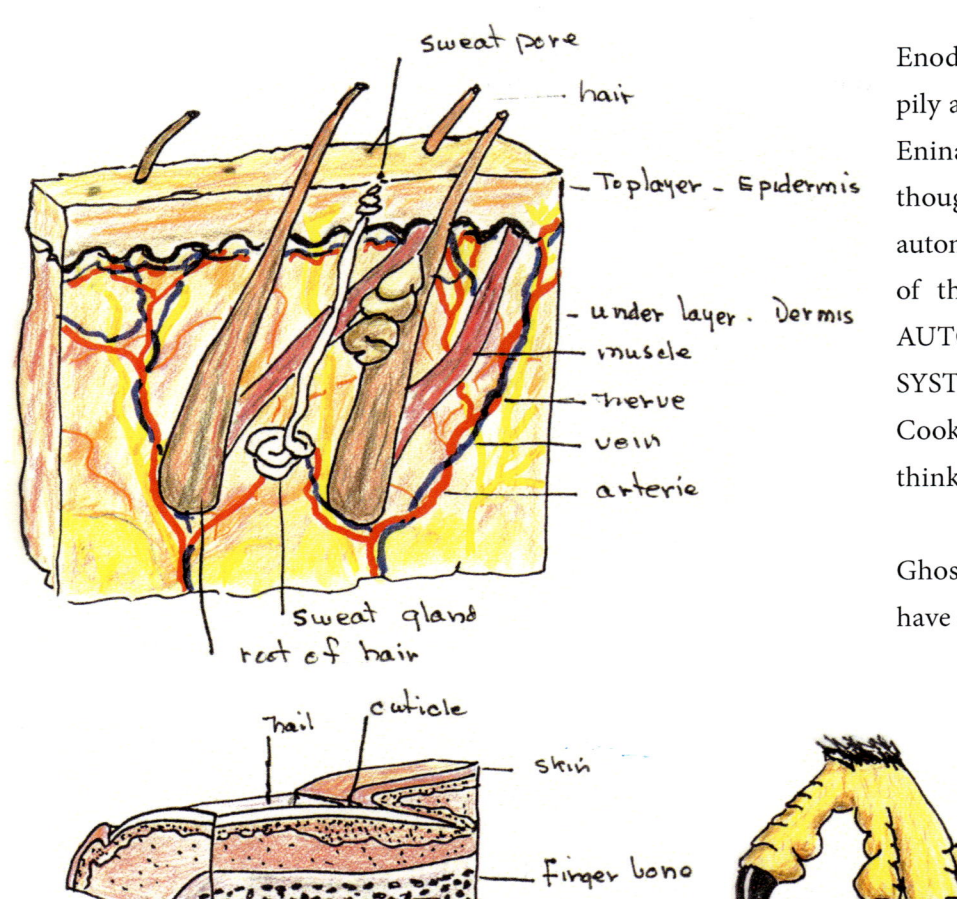

Enod Ton was munching happily and dropping crumbs (which Eninac was eating). After some thought he said, "All of this is automatic? I know which part of the body controls that. The AUTONOMIC NERVOUS SYSTEM! There, Ghost Host. Cookies DO help with my thinking."

Ghost Host sighed. Maybe I better have a cookie.

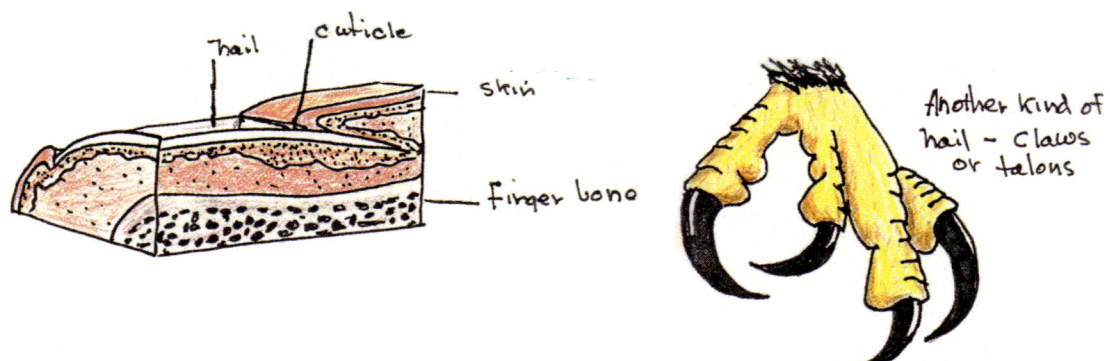

"Look Ghost Host, I have found a drawing of the skin. Whoa! All of that is skin? It looks like a subway system with poles."

Your descriptions are always good, Enod Ton. Poles, indeed. Those are hairs.

"Hairs. Of course. Hairs do grow in the skin."

They not only grow IN the skin, they ARE skin.

"I am boggled. Hair is skin! Next you will tell me that nails are skin."

Enod Ton, you have mystic powers. Nails are skin, too.

Enod Ton was quiet, but only for a few seconds. "Ghost Host, you must know that this is almost too much for me. Let me review this. There are different kinds of skin: the kind all over the body, hair and nails."

That is totally correct, which brings us to the second layer of skin. The hair grows from the second layer, as do the nails. Look at the drawing of the skin. See where the hair starts?

Enod Ton was so involved in looking at the drawing that he did not say one word. Ghost Host thought there was a slight sound that meant, "yes".

There are sweat glands there, too, and blood vessels, and nerves.

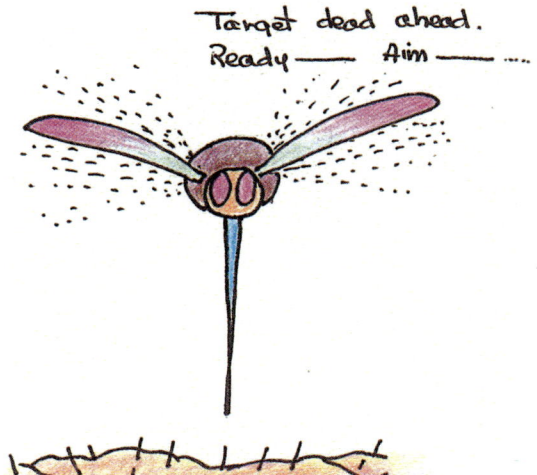

"Nerves! That is so that we know when we have touched something, or something is too hot. Now I see what you mean when you say that the skin protects us."

Enod Ton, I almost always know what I am talking about. That's why it is fun being a ghost. Since no one can see me, people don't know where to look for me to disagree.

"I don't know where you are but I can see the grass move".

Let's get on with the skin. There are some 'fun' things you might want to know.

"Fun things are the ones I like the best, Ghost Host."

We will start with the skin. You are shedding skin all of the time. The outer layer drops off and makes room for a fresh layer.

"No, no, no, Ghost Host. Like a snake or a lizard? I refuse to shed my skin. I do not even have it yet and you are talking about my losing it."

You don't have a choice, Enod Ton. It is what healthy skin does. All that is lost is replaced by the cells underneath.

"Oh. Well, in that case it's OK. What else about the skin?"

Goodness! I forgot to mention bitsy things like mosquitoes. One more very necessary thing. Your skin has all sorts of nerves under the top layer. These nerves tell you five things: touch, pain, heat, cold and pressure. All of these are for protection of your body. Do you remember talking about these?

"I remember them from our chapter about SENSORS. What else, Ghost Host?"

I might mention itching. Watch the mosquitoes! Now we have the hair. There are two color chemicals that make all hair color. They are dark brown and red. The mixing of the two colors gives various shades and colors. Color is usually inherited from your parents.

"The person who makes me a whole person will give me hair color. I am looking forward to that. Are there any other 'hair facts?"

On the body, where does hair NOT grow?

"I never thought of that. Are there places with no hair?"

Yes, several. The palms of your hands, soles of your feet, lips and eyelids have no hair.

"That makes sense but there is hair on the eyelids."

Those are eyelashes and are only on the very edge of the lids. They are very sensitive and protect the eyes.

Will Eninac have all of this?

He will have a lot of it. He will even have eyelashes. His eyes will be a little different because he won't see color. His ears will hear better and his sense of smell are far better than humans'.

Eninac rattled around and wagged his tail violently to let Enod Ton and Ghost Host know that he had heard about his new body. Ghost Host thought he saw him smiling.

"We see things on TV about changing color of hair and nails and even skin. Is there any part of the body where the color cannot be changed?"

There is, Enod Ton. We cannot change the color of our eyes. They are what we call "forever". You have reminded me of something I would have

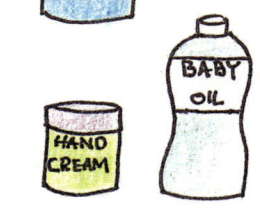

forgotten. Our skin is sensitive to the sunrays. It will change color just by being out in the light. If you are out too long, your skin will burn.

"Uh - oh. That sounds like it is not a healthy thing to do. I will be careful, Ghost Host."

Well, Enod Ton, since we are almost finished with our BODY HOUSE, I know you must have something to say.

"Yes, I do, Ghost Host. Now I can use lots of wonderful hand lotion. Some of it smells like vanilla wafers. It all smells so good."

Ghost Host laughed so hard that sitting down was best. Eninac woofed three times and wagged his tail in circles.

DECISION TIME

"Now Student Guests, it is time for you to decide what Eninac and I will be. We are very excited about our new lives.

Not only do you need to put us together, you will have to decide on all of the things listed below: You will need a piece of paper to write down all of the things you want us to be. We are very anxious to know who we will be and what we will be. Please make us the new Enod Ton and Eninac"

For ENOD TON	for ENINAC
Girl or boy	male or female
Short, medium, tall	small. medium, big
Hair color	coat color
Eye color	long or short hair
Special abilities	special abilities

And anything else you can think of.

NEW NAME _____ NEW NAME _____

"Now that you have decided about all of the things in the list above, take a piece of your favorite drawing paper and draw the new Enod Ton and Eninac. Don't forget our new names."

Woof, woooof, woof.

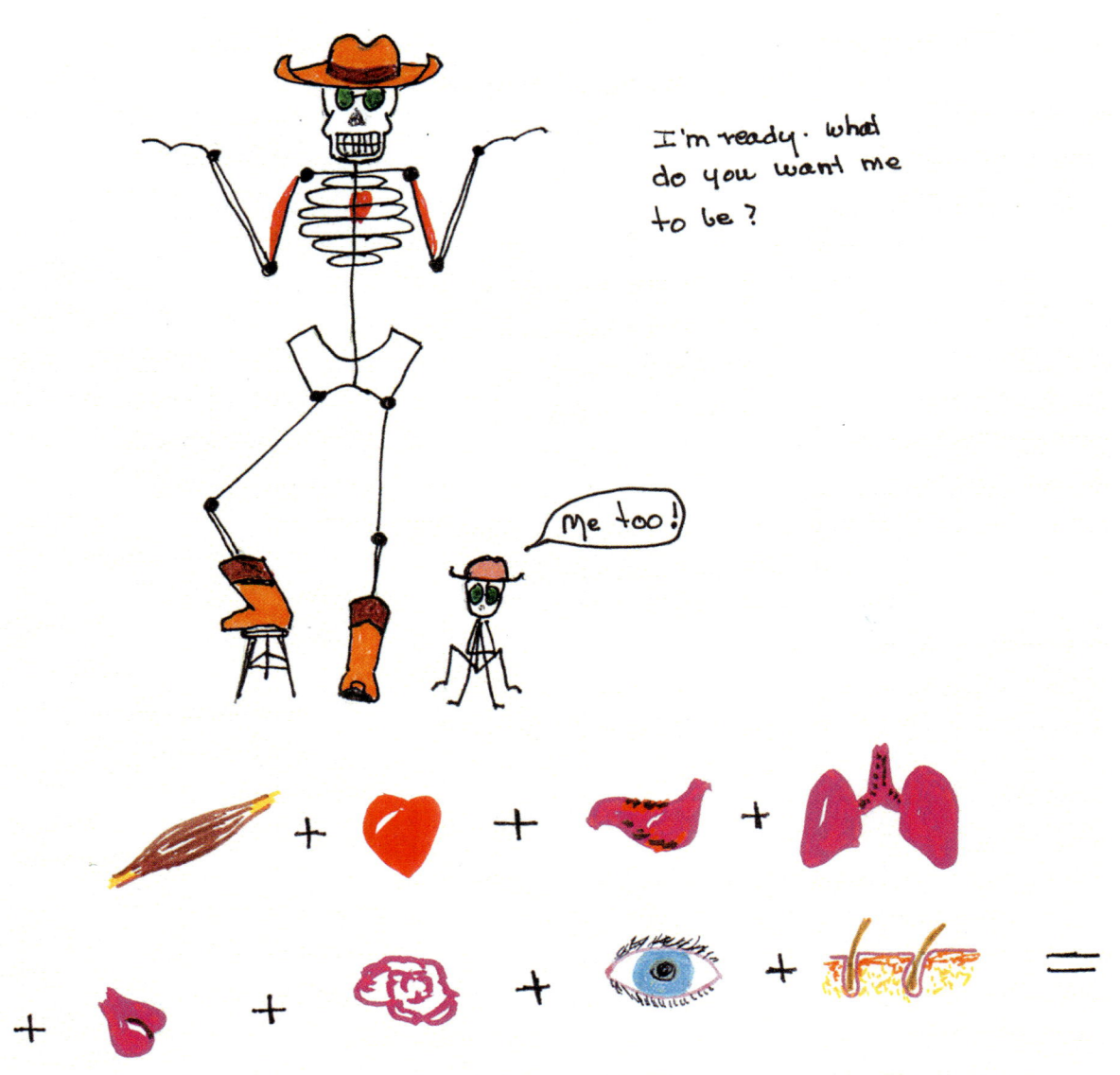

THANK YOU, STUDENT GUESTS
AN END AND A BEGINNING

This is a SAD-GLAD time for us, Enod Ton. We have come to the end of our trip through the BODY HOUSE. Very soon now, you will be a complete person. Eninac will be a complete dog. That will be a new beginning for you both.

Enod Ton did not answer. Eninac lay quietly in the grass. Everything was still except the ducks quacking on the lake.

After a few minutes, Enod Ton said "I have waited a very long time for this day, Ghost Host. Now I am not sure that I want to leave our movable classroom and the cookies and your car. Mostly, I don't want to say goodbye to you."

Enod Ton, (you won't have that name much longer), this is a wonderful time for you. A new name, you will be a girl or boy, a new family. What a great day!

"Everything you say is true, Ghost Host. You have been a good friend. When my good friend goes away, it will leave a hole in my life. Can Eninac and I come to see you? Well, that was a foolish question! We have never seen you. But you know what I mean."

Eninac raised his head and wagged his tail slightly.

Of course you can come to "see" me. I will always welcome you and Eninac. Remember, I may not recognize the "new you", but I will know your voice and your funny dance steps.

Enod Ton was feeling better. "That's right, Ghost Host. How would you recognize either of us? We shall dance and sing all the way to your house, just so you will know us."

Eninac was frolicking about in the grass, wildly wagging his tail and woofing a lot.

Oh Dear! Another dance. On that, I had better leave. I will not say 'good bye', Enod Ton. I will say 'I'll see you around'".

Enod Ton and Eninac watched Ghost Host's car roar away in a cloud of rust.

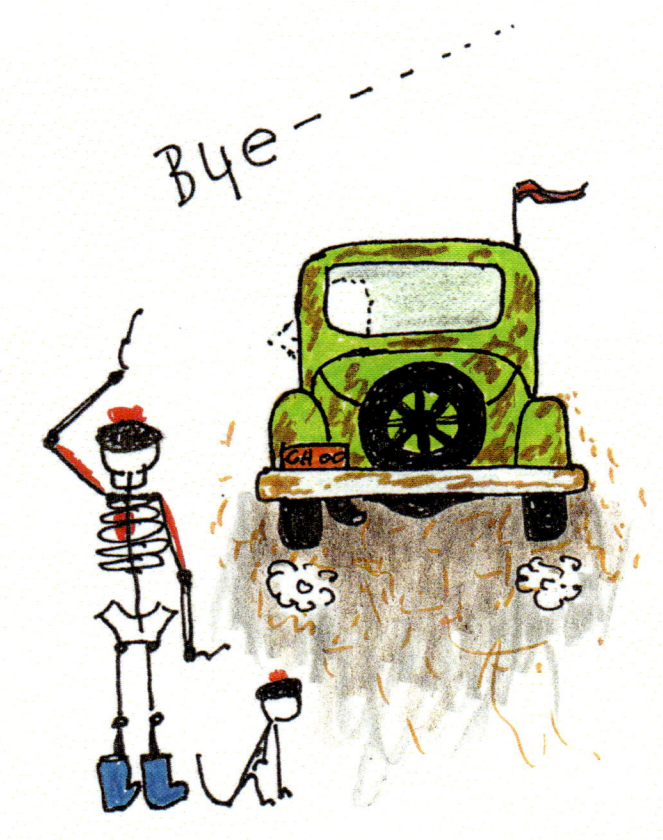

THE BODY HOUSE ARCHITECT

Any attempts at writing were nebulous, embryonic efforts, born on smoky, noisy troop trains in the unforgettable wartime '40's. Everyone was either saying frantically happy "hellos" or soul rending "good byes". I did both and tried to get those moments on paper. The recorded emotions stayed with me for a while, but like most all duffel bags, were lost.

War ended and education took precedent. Writing had to be channeled into educational survival efforts. There were research papers to be done, thesis research to be written with strict formality and reports from the physiology lab to be submitted.

The next opportunity to write was new course outlines and content to help shape and guide the young minds. The famous "Nine Year Plan" developed. With university teaching in mind, the plan was to work with elementary age children for three years, middle school for three years, high school, three years. With that broad experience, I felt ready to shape older minds.

It never happened. I fell in love with the little ones and stayed four years. Already behind, I survived middle school age kids by having a sense of humor and thinking of them as "exposed glands". High school, college-bound seniors became the passion of the years. In the process of writing a new curriculum for them in physiological psychology, I included an extended unit on preteen growth and development. It was during this era that I began thinking about a fun book about the body for little people. Thus, Enod Ton, Ghost Host and Eninac were born. They became family.

Retirement has given me time and securities to have the luxury of letting the above three ramble about in my head, making it eventually to paper. When they had completed their journey and we said goodbye, I will admit to some tears. We completed our journey together in January 1997. I hope we meet again.
Margaret Lawrence

WORKBOOK

Hi – MY name is Enod Ton.

Welcome to the Body House. As you can see, I am missing a few things. Don't worry. As we travel through the body house, I will collect all of the equipment I need to be complete. Am I male or female? I don't know yet. Let's examine what I have, then we'll know what I need. Refer to your book to help me find the answers to what I already have in the way of a body.

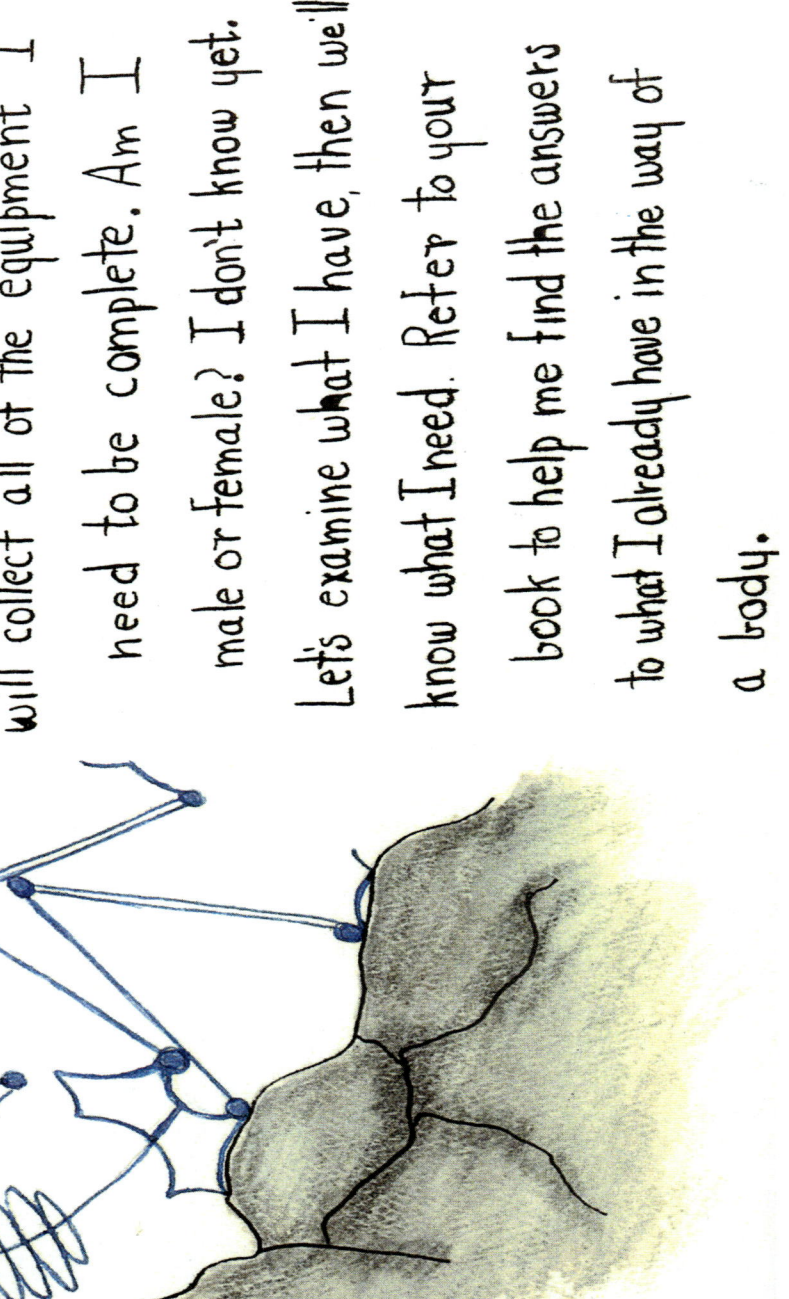

CONTENTS

I. Framing – Skeleton
II. Siding – Muscle
III. Intercommunication – Heart & Circulation *(conveyer)*
IV. The Kitchen – Digestion
V. Ventilation – Respiration
VI. Maintenance – Glands
VII. Electrical System – Nerves
VIII. The Computer – Brain
IX. Sensors – Senses
X. Rebuilding – Reproduction

1. How many bones are there in the body? _____
2. There are two main jobs the skeleton does. What are these? _____
3. The system of bones which allow us to stand upright is called _____.
4. How many bones are there in question #3? _____
5. What do we find between each vertebrae? _____

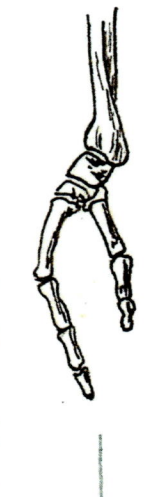

6. The most important part of the whole body is the brain. What bone structure protects it? _____
7. The vertebral column protects a very vital organ. What is it? _____
8. Surrounding our lungs, and acting as a bellows are bones called _____. How many total do you have? _____ There are 7 pairs called _____ and 5 pairs called _____.

9. You are holding a pencil or pen. Bones are basic in making this possible.
How many bones are there in your arm, wrist, hand and fingers?

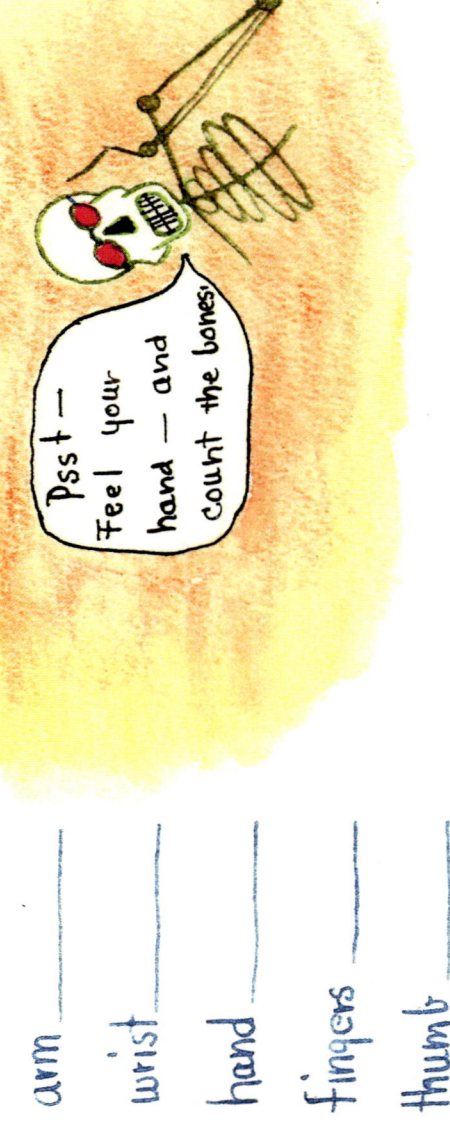

arm _____
wrist _____
hand _____
fingers _____
thumb _____

10. The largest, strongest bone in the body is called the _____.
This bone is located where? _____

11. The body bends at the joints. Test your fingers. Will they bend backward?
What kind of a joint is this? Name one other joint like this.

12. There are three other kinds of joints; pivot, gliding and ball-and-socket.
Could you tell where each is found?

3

13. Bones are held together at the joints by white glue. No? Well, what then? _____

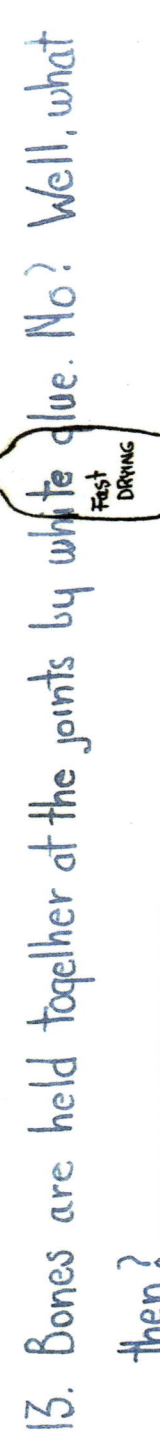

14. Oil lubricates an automobile engine. Our joints need lubrication too. What do we call this fluid? _____

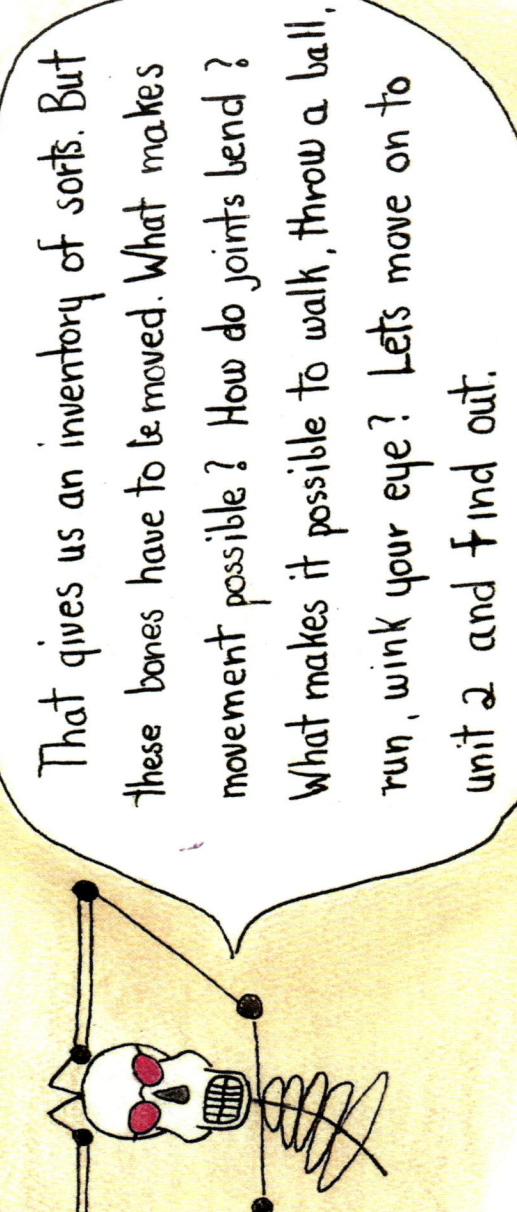

That gives us an inventory of sorts. But these bones have to be moved. What makes movement possible? How do joints bend? What makes it possible to walk, throw a ball, run, wink your eye? Lets move on to unit 2 and find out.

Siding ~ Muscle 2

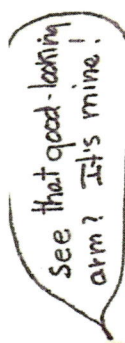

"See that good-lookin arm? It's mine!"

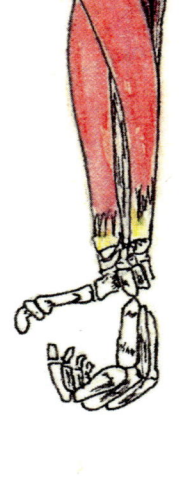

1. How are muscles anchored to the bones?
2. Nerve impulses flow continuously to the muscles from……?
3. What happens when the nerve to the muscle is cut?
4. Is it true that your muscles give your body form?
5. Your muscles are in a constant state of readiness and partially contracted. This is called……?
6. Two factors determine muscle growth and strength. These are …… + ……
7. What one factor has most influence on body type?
8. When a muscle contracts does it get longer or shorter?

Siding - 2

9. The muscles that bend a joint of the body are called _____, while those that straighten the joints are called _____.

10. Which of the following does not belong in the group?
skeletal, smooth, striated

11. Overuse of muscles cause a build-up of what in the muscles?

12. When you puff and pant after exercise, this is due to _____.

13. Muscles which form thin sheets of tissue are called....?

14. Lack of oxygen to a muscle will cause the muscle to _____.

15. What is a bruise?

16. Muscles contract in response to stimuli from the brain. There are three other types of stimuli which make muscles contract. Name these.

17. Which type of muscle tires slowly?

Intercommunication ~ Heart and Circulation 3

1. Is your heart the center of your emotions? _____
   Does your heart fall in love? _____
2. What is the basic function of your heart? _____
3. Which side of the heart pumps dark red de-oxygenated blood? _____; bright red oxygenated? _____
4. Where does the blood go from the left side of the heart? _____; right side? _____.

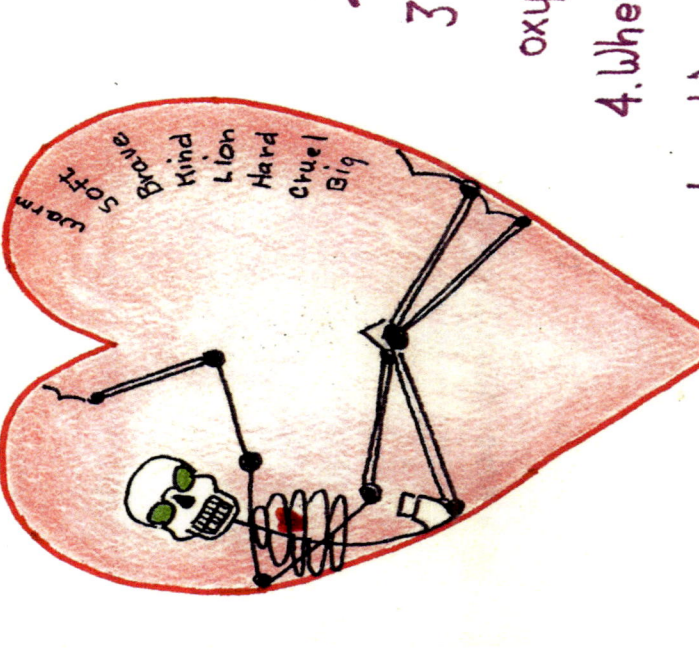

5. The upper chambers of the heart are called _____ while the lower chambers of the heart are called _____.
6. Circulation within the walls of the heart is called _____
7. Which walls are the strongest, auricles or ventricles? _____

Intercom 2

8. Name the sections which are numbered in the drawing.

9. Using arrows, draw the direction the blood flows through the heart. Remember, there are "two hearts".

10. What is the "heart beat"?

11. What is the largest artery in the body? What is the largest vein?

12. What is the smallest branch of the arteries?

13. Where does the blood give up the carbon dioxide and pick up oxygen?

14. If the blood is cut off to tissue, what happens?

15. What is the other circulatory system?

16. Arteriosclerosis is another word for what?

17. How many miles of blood vessels do you have?

18. Which blood vessels carry the blood to the heart?...... Away from the heart?.....

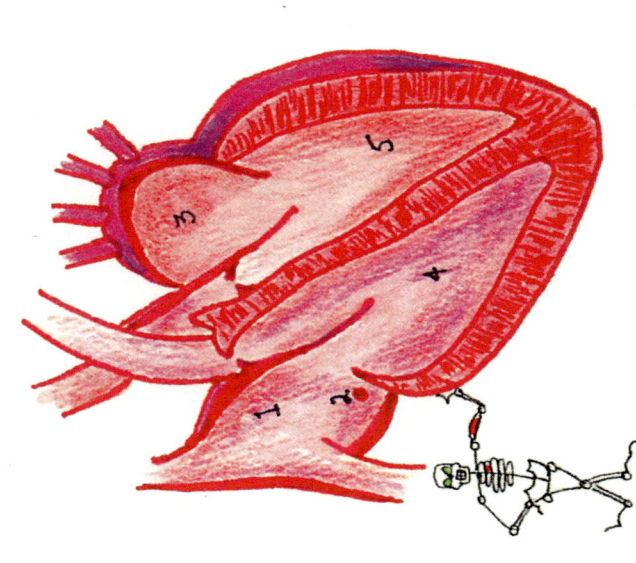

19. What prevents the blood from flowing backward?

20. What sets the pace of the heart?

21. What is another name for the answer in question 20?

22. The average adult heartbeat is _____ per minute.

23. There are two places in which blood is stored while you are at rest. These are _____ and _____.

24. For an average adult under 40, blood pressure is about _____.

25. Which is the most serious, high or low blood pressure?

26. How do all of the cells in the body communicate with each other?

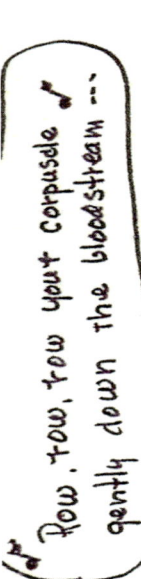

Ventilation ~ Respiration 5

1. How do the following living things breathe? Fish, earthworm, grasshopper, a leaf.

2. Can a fish drown?

3. Supposing you put a fish into boiled (and cooled) water. Could it breathe?

4. Which lung is larger? Which lung is longer? How many lobes does each have?

5. You are flying at 8000 meters in a hot air balloon. You are feeling weak, slightly paralyzed, and unable to move your tongue. What is the problem?

6. The release of energy for life and living is called what?

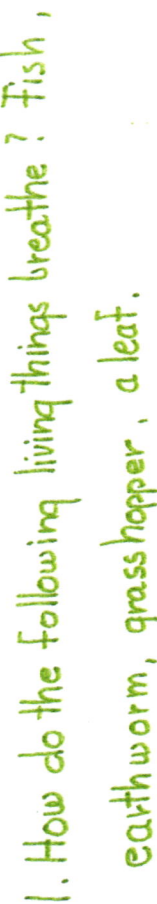

Ventilation 2

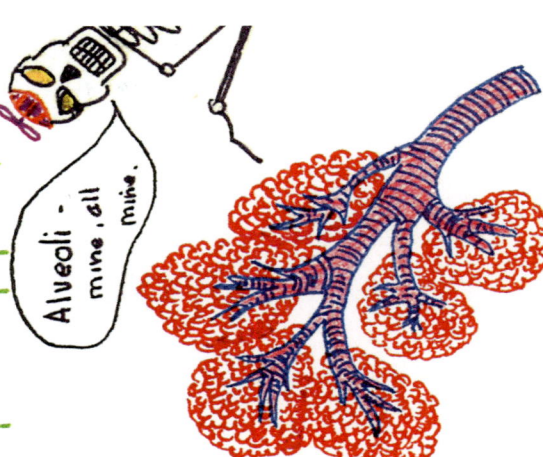

"Alveoli - mine, all mine."

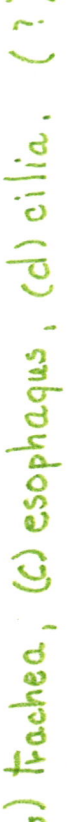

$C_6H_{12}O_6 + 6O_2 + 6CO_2 + 6H_2O + E = HE$
All that to blow up this balloon. It boggles the mind.

7. Is the larynx part of the (a) bronchial tubes, (b) trachea, (c) esophagus, (d) cilia. (?)

8. Which one of the following is not in the chest
(a) trachea, (b) bronchi, (c) lungs, (d) larynx. (?)

9. Air must be processed before it reaches the lungs. The _____ warms and moistens it. _____ filters out dust and the _____.

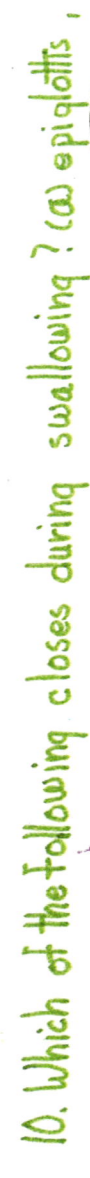

10. Which of the following closes during swallowing? (a) epiglottis, (b) esophagus, (c) larynx, (d) trachea.

11. The place where air from the nose and food from the mouth cross the same path is called the _____?

12. When you strum a guitar the strings vibrate. Your vocal cords vibrate when you exhale. When the cords are tight are the tones high or low? How many cords are there?

Ventilation 3

13. What is the "Adams apple"?
14. Why are men's voices deeper?
15. Which muscle controls breathing?
16. Everything has a control center. Where is the breathing center?
17. The rate of breathing depends upon the CO_2 level in the blood. How can this level be lowered?
18. Sudden sharp contractions of the diaphragm are called ....
19. The lungs are made up of millions of air sacs called ....
20. Why is one lung larger than the other?
21. Is the process of breathing mechanical or chemical?
22. Is talking done when you inhale or exhale?
23. What is laryngitis?

THE KITCHEN ~ DIGESTION 4

1. What five areas make up the alimentary canal?

2. Most peoples alimentary canal is about ____ times as long as the body.

3. Digestion goes on in which three parts of the alimentary canal?

4. Food particles are broken down chemically by ....?

5. The salivary glands are located where?

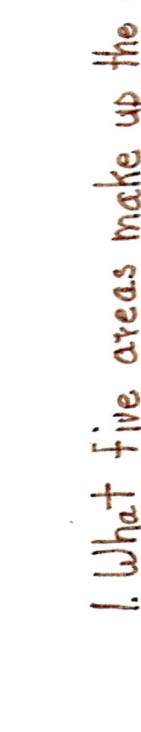

6. These salivary glands make how much saliva every day?

7. How does the food move through the digestive tract?

8. The stomach is a muscular pouch which holds how much?

9. The gastric juice is made up of pepsin which begins digestion of ____ and hydrochloric acid which does several things. Name three.

Kitchen 2

10. Why doesn't pepsin digest the stomach itself?
11. The valve at the end of the stomach is called ....
12. About how long is the small intestine?
13. What holds the small intestine in place?
14. Where does the majority of digestion take place?
15. There are three pancreatic enzymes below. Tell what each digests ① pancreatic amylase, ② trypsin, ③ pancreatic lipase + bile.

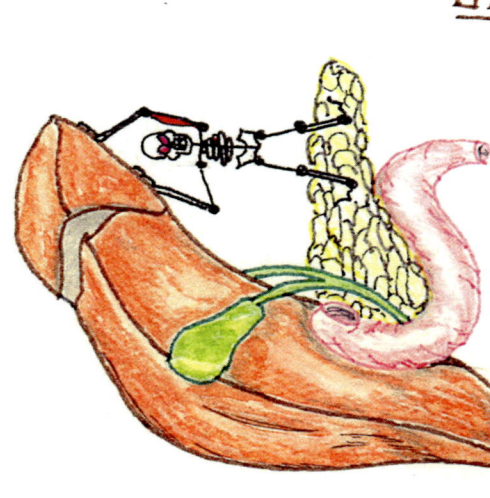

16. There are tiny projectiles in the small intestine. These are called .... What is the function of these projectiles?
17. What is the chief work of the large intestine?
18. What is the name of the pouch at the end of the large intestine?
19. Where is the appendix located?
20. Which two vitamins are not destroyed by cooking?

Well, we have come through 5 units. I seem to have picked up a few items. I don't think these items are particularly pretty - but they are necessary. I really don't want to be Enad Ton forever. You are going to give me a name in 5 more units.

Now, you and I both know there are many missing parts. Hopefully I will acquire the rest of what I need in the next 5 units. Meanwhile, meet my friend Eninac. This critter needs parts too. Perhaps we can be of help. Let's move on and see what happens.

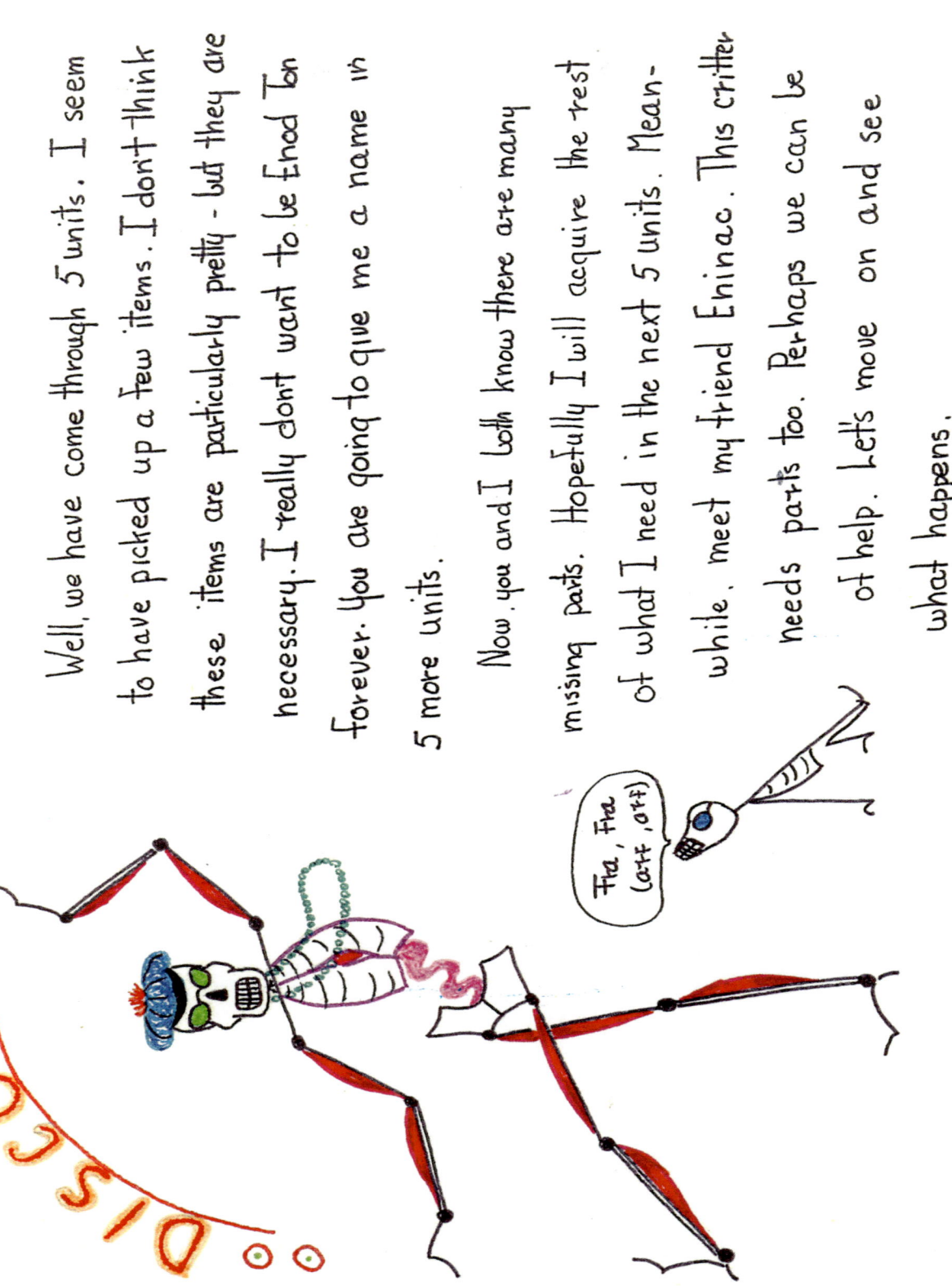

ELECTRICAL SYSTEM — NERVES

1. There are three related nervous systems. Can you name these?
2. The cells of the nervous system are called _____.
3. A nerve impulse is what kind of a change in the nerve cell?
4. There are three kinds of neurons. Name these and tell what they do.
5. Do the associative neurons make up the gray or white matter?
6. The fibers in a nerve vary in size. The (thinest, thickest) fibers transmit at 3-4 feet per second. The (thinest, thickest) fibers transmit at 450 ft. per second.
7. The fast neurons transmit to (closest, fartherest) parts of the body.
8. Which nerves carry information from the sensory organs to the brain?

Electrical system

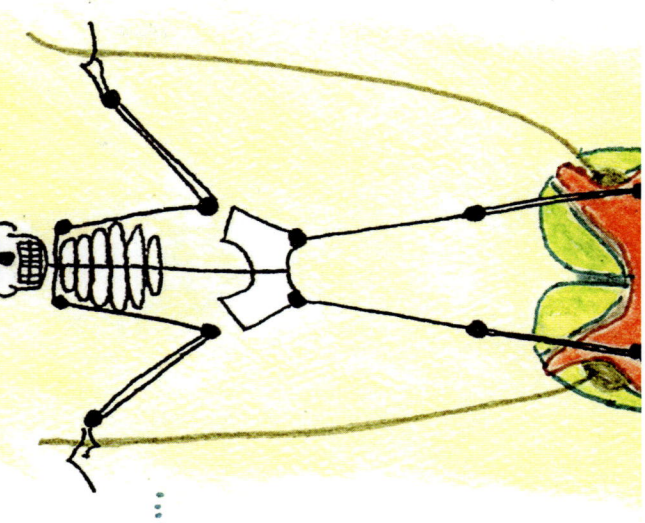

... nerves extend outward from the brain while the ..... nerves come
ly from the spinal cord.

... nerves carry orders from the central nervous system to the muscles?

... nerve carries sensory messages from the eye to the brain?

plicated neural relay station is generally called a ....

utonomic nervous system controls functions which
(voluntary, involuntary).

o subdivisions of the autonomic N.S. are ..... & ....

u have any control over your autonomic N.S.?

s the most simple level of nerve action?

part of the nervous system is the "quiet" part?

he axon of one cell lies close to the dendrites
next cell, this is called a ....

Electrical system 3

98

THE COMPUTER ~ BRAIN (and spinal cord)

1. The central nervous system is composed of .... and ....
2. What boney structures protect the brain and spinal cord?
3. The membranes protecting the spinal cord are called........
4. What is the name of the fluid which protects the cord?

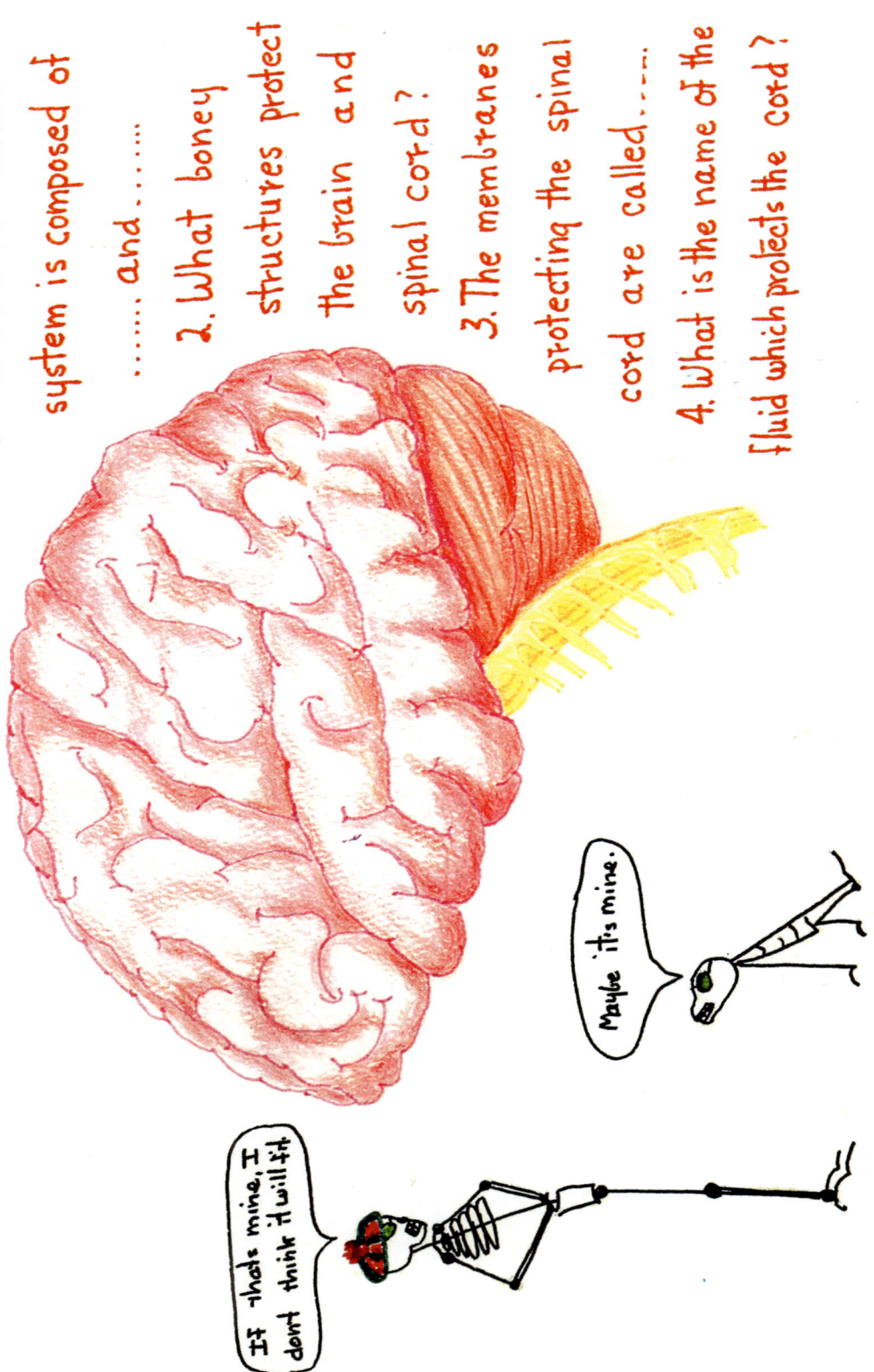

"Maybe it's mine."

"If that's mine, I don't think it will fit."

Computer 2

5. The largest part of the brain is called ....
6. The surface of the largest part of the brain is called ....
7. The folds on the surface of the cerebrum are called ....
8. The motor area of the brain controls what function?
9. If you are right handed, which side of the brain controls what function?
10. Which part of the brain contains learning?
11. Which part of the brain coordinates muscle activity?
12. There are two brain sections which are concerned with body temperature and connections. What are these?

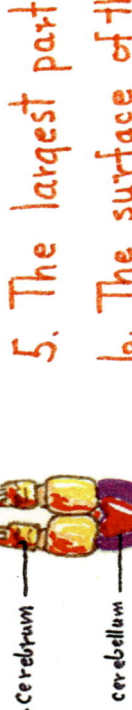
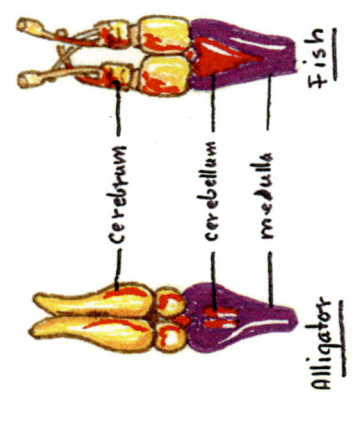
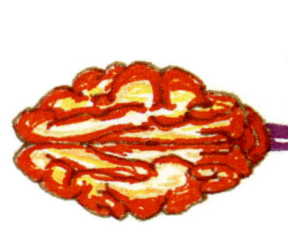
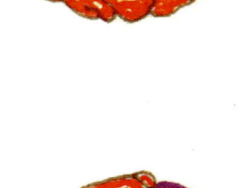
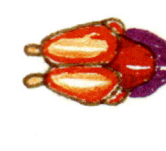
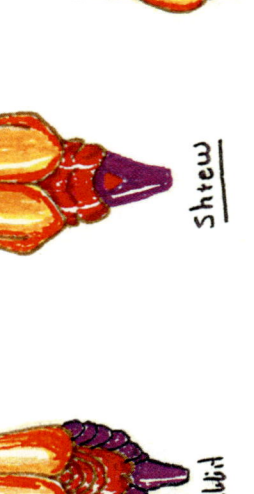

Computer 3

13. Breathing, heart action, digestion, to mention a few, are controlled in which area?

14. The pathway for sensory and motor nerves is located where?

15. On the drawing below identify the parts of the brain.

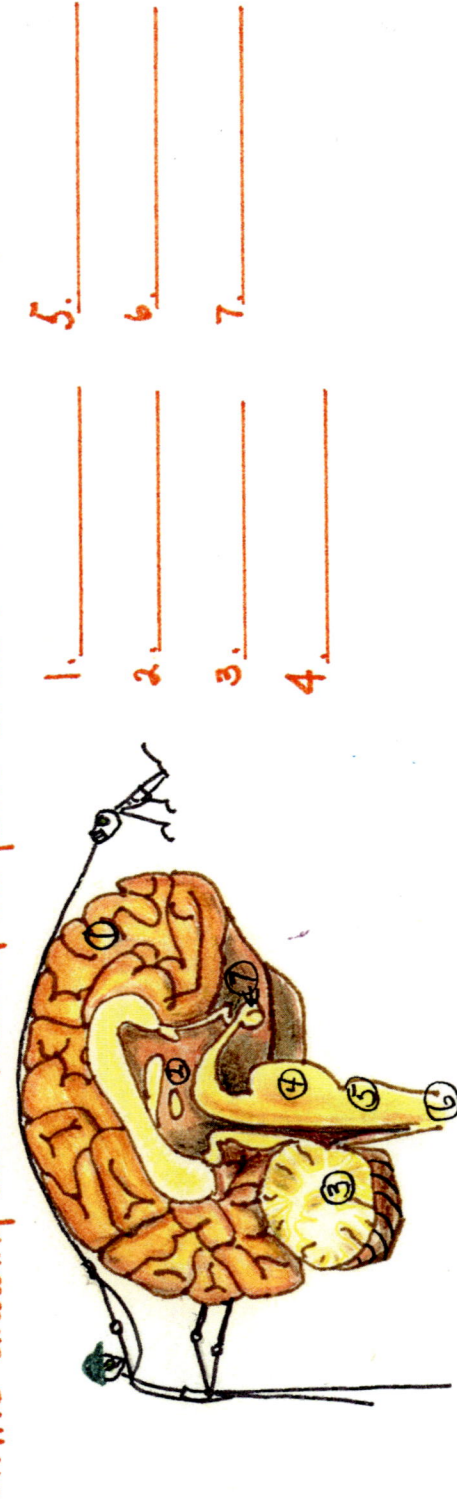

1. _____
2. _____
3. _____
4. _____
5. _____
6. _____
7. _____

16. On the drawing below you will find numbered areas. Identify these areas.

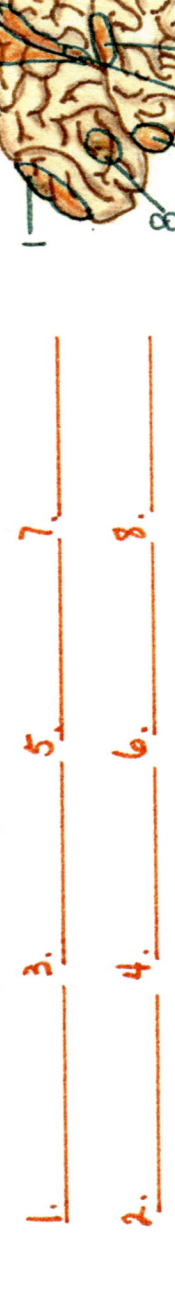

1. _____
2. _____
3. _____
4. _____
5. _____
6. _____
7. _____
8. _____

101

Computer 4

17. Because the brain is so complex, we need to understand all we can. Below is a list of functions. Can you tell which part of the brain is involved?

a. thinking _____
b. reasoning _____
c. body well being _____
d. water need _____
e. pons + cerebellum connection _____
f. consciousness _____
g. body temperature _____
h. connects brain stem and cerebrum _____
i. heart control _____
j. speech _____
k. posture _____
l. breathing _____
m. swimming _____
n. perception _____

"Hang in there, baby."

Sensors — Senses

1. What is the difference between an oculist and an ophthalmologist? Is an optometrist a doctor? Can he perscribe glasses? Does an optician perscribe medicine? Exactly what does he do?

2. Name the white, outer, protective layer of the eye.

3. The dark middle layer of the eye which carries most of the blood vessels is called what?

4. Which is the light sensitive part of the eye?

5. Which part of the sclera is transparent?

6. What type of cells make up the pupil?

Sensors 2

7. Where is the color of the eyes located?
8. A part of the eye adjusts to light. What is it?
9. Which main part of the eye lies behind the pupil?
10. The lens adjusts to distances. This process is called what?
11. Which humor gives shape to the eyeball?
12. There are two kinds of light sensitive cells. These are ...... and ......
13. The spot of most acute vision on the retina is called what?
14. The spot where there are no rods and cones is called what?
15. A deficiency of which vitamin causes "night blindness"?
16. The type of vision using both eyes is called what?
17. The image at which you are looking is upside down on the retina. Which part of the eye caused this?

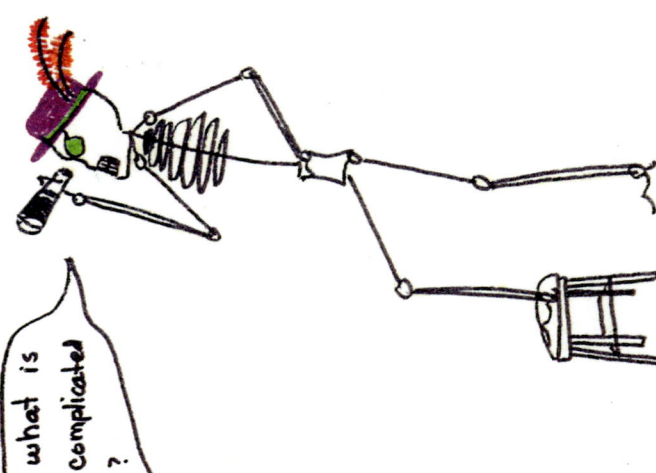

"Now what is that complicated mess?"

18. On the drawing below, identify the numbered parts.

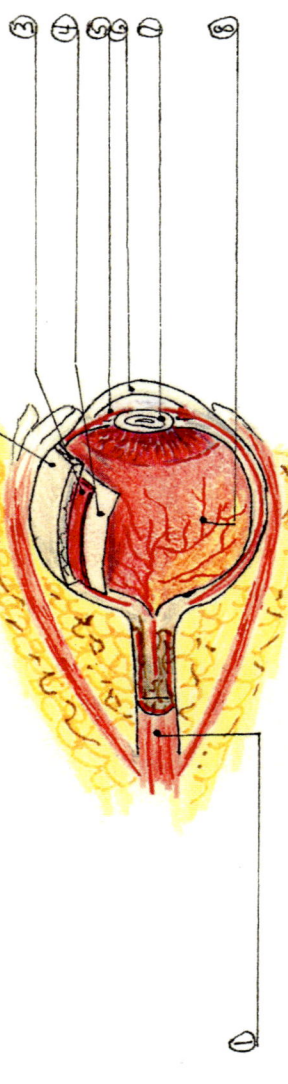

19. What instrument is used to measure hearing?
20. A medical doctor who specializes in treatment of the ear is called ....
21. Name the three parts of the ear.
22. What is the tympanic membrane?
23. The middle ear and the throat are connected by what?
24. Which part of the inner ear is essential to balance?   Why?
25. Is there sound on the moon?
26. Which nerve carries sound vibrations to the brain?

Senses 4

27. Will listening to loud sounds for a period of time damage your hearing?
28. Which organs in the ell tell you that you are standing upright?
29. Identify the parts of the ear which are numbered in the drawing.

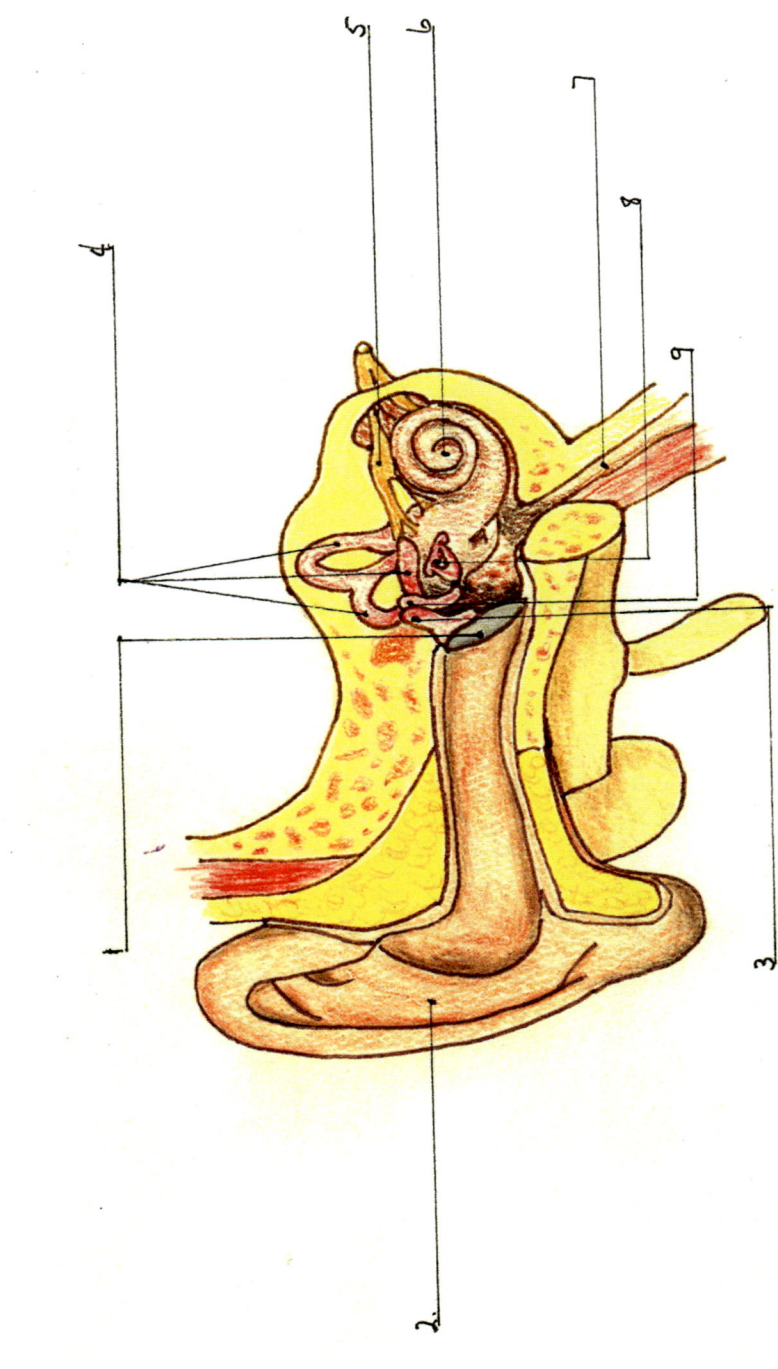

106

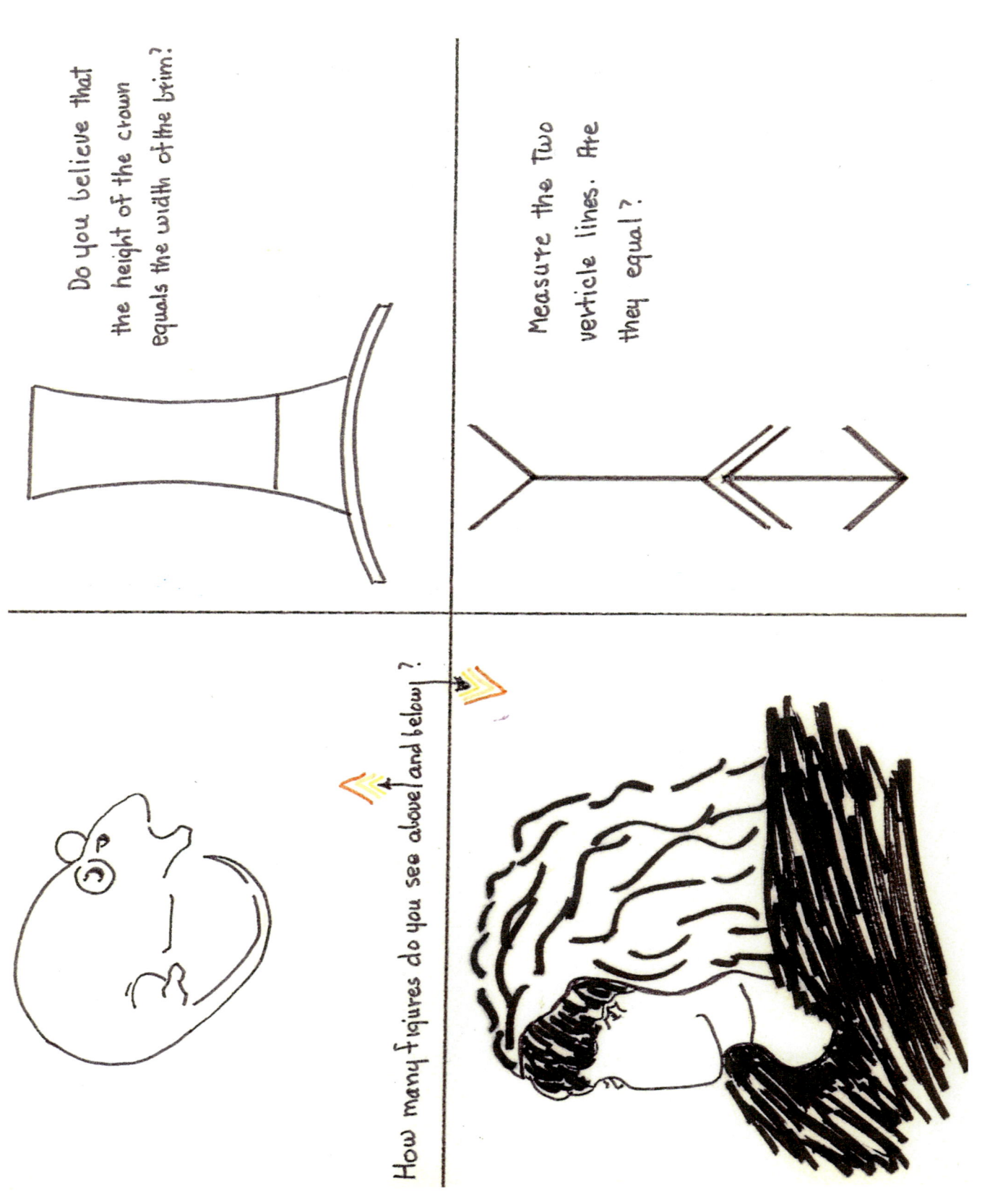

Blind spot: Close your left eye. Stare at X with right eye. Move card toward you until dot disappears.

Necker Cube: Look at it for a few moments and see if you can change the planes.

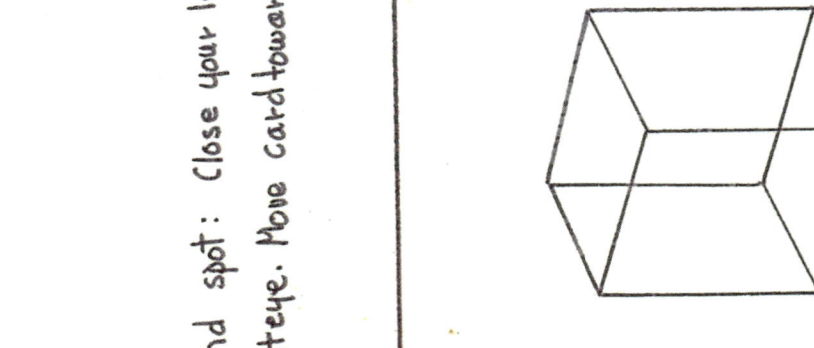

open

How many figures do you see?

d. Somatotrophic harmone has to do with what?

e. The harmone which has to do with producing milk in the mammary glands.

7. Which harmone controls blood sugar level?

8. Where is the above harmone produced?

9. The gland which controls the metabolism is what?

10. You start across the street at a crosswalk. A car does not stop as it should. You jump back. Where did you get the sudden energy?

11. Secretin is the harmone for what?

12. The following body functions occur under the control of which particular gland?

a. extra energy
b. weight
c. sperm
d. sugar breakdown
e. iodine
f. ovum

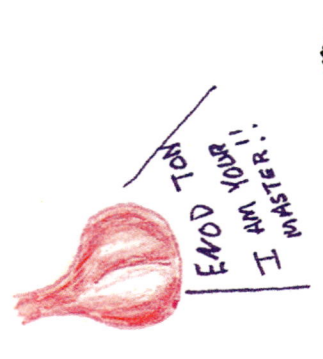

ENOD TOM
I AM YOUR
MASTER!!

Yes, oh great one.
I hear you

Maintenance 3

g. calcium
h. puberty changes
i. ATCH
j. body's immunization
k. inhibits sexual development
l. dwarfism
m. giantism
n. goiter

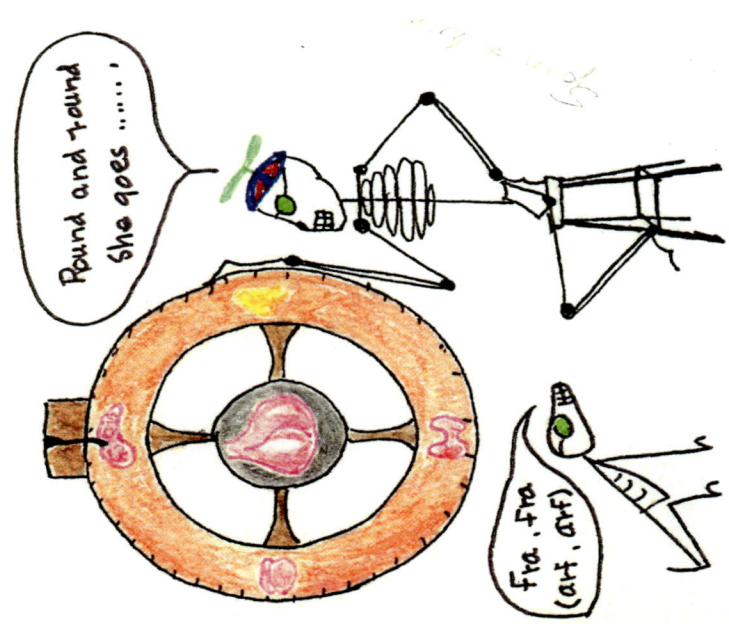

Problem: Jean's clothes have become too tight. Tom's voice slides up and down. Dan's arms seem too long. Laura's interests are changing. Explain why all of the above events are happening.

Rebuilding — Reproduction 10

> Well, this is our 10th unit. When we finish this one my body will be complete. You are going to have to make a decision. Am I going to be male or female? My name is still Enod Ion I am hoping for a new name, one to fit my sex. And what about Enviac? That's another decision for you. Let's go through the questions below, and when you have completed them you will find "a decision section".

Names: Tobias, Harry, Daphine, Iris, Lionel, Mona, Edwina, Alberta, Clyde, Terence, Sean, Evan, Olivia, Horace, Aliza, Percy, Gregory, Irene, Basil, Sonja, Freda, Elsa, Elmer

1. Are the ovaries found in the male or female?

2. Are the testes found in the male or female?

3. The process of physical changes into adulthood is called ………

4. Which gland begins the changes in the ovaries and testes?

5. What is the major male hormone? Is this found in women?

Rebuilding 2

6. When body hair begins to grow and voices change, these characteristics are called what?

7. What is the major female harmone? Is this found in men?

8. When the ovaries release a mature egg once a month, this is called what?

9. When the lining of the uterus is shed, this is called ....

10. How many days from the beginning of menstruation to the next?

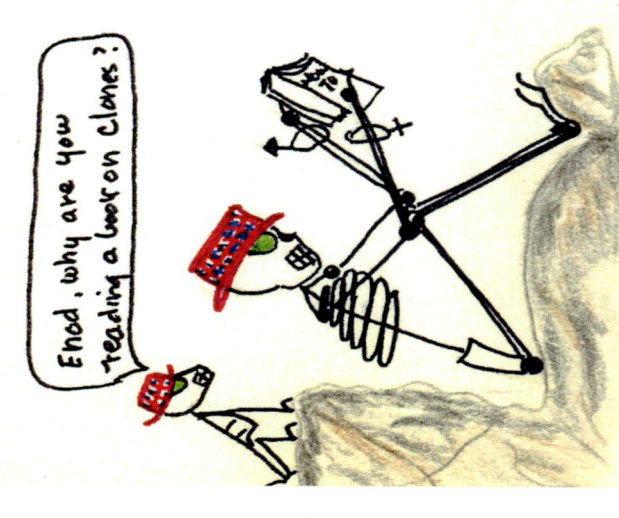

11. About how many days after menstruation begins does ovulation occur?

12. What do the testes make other than harmones?

13. Name the 2 main organs of reproduction of the female.

14. Name the 2 main organs of reproduction of the male.

15. IN the female, part of the body opens to the outside. Name this reproductive part.

Rebuilding 3

16. When the ovum and sperm come together, this is called ………

17. The fertilized ovum moves down the uterine tube and plants itself where?

18. The fertilized ovum is called _____ until the end of the 2nd month. It is then called _____ until birth.

19. Gestation takes how many days for the following:

a. mouse _____
b. dog _____
c. cat _____
d. pig _____
e. monkey _____
f. man _____
g. horse _____
h. elephant _____

20. Identical twins form from ___ ova and ___ sperm. Fraternal twins form from ___ ova and ___ sperm.

21. Is there such a thing as identical triplets?

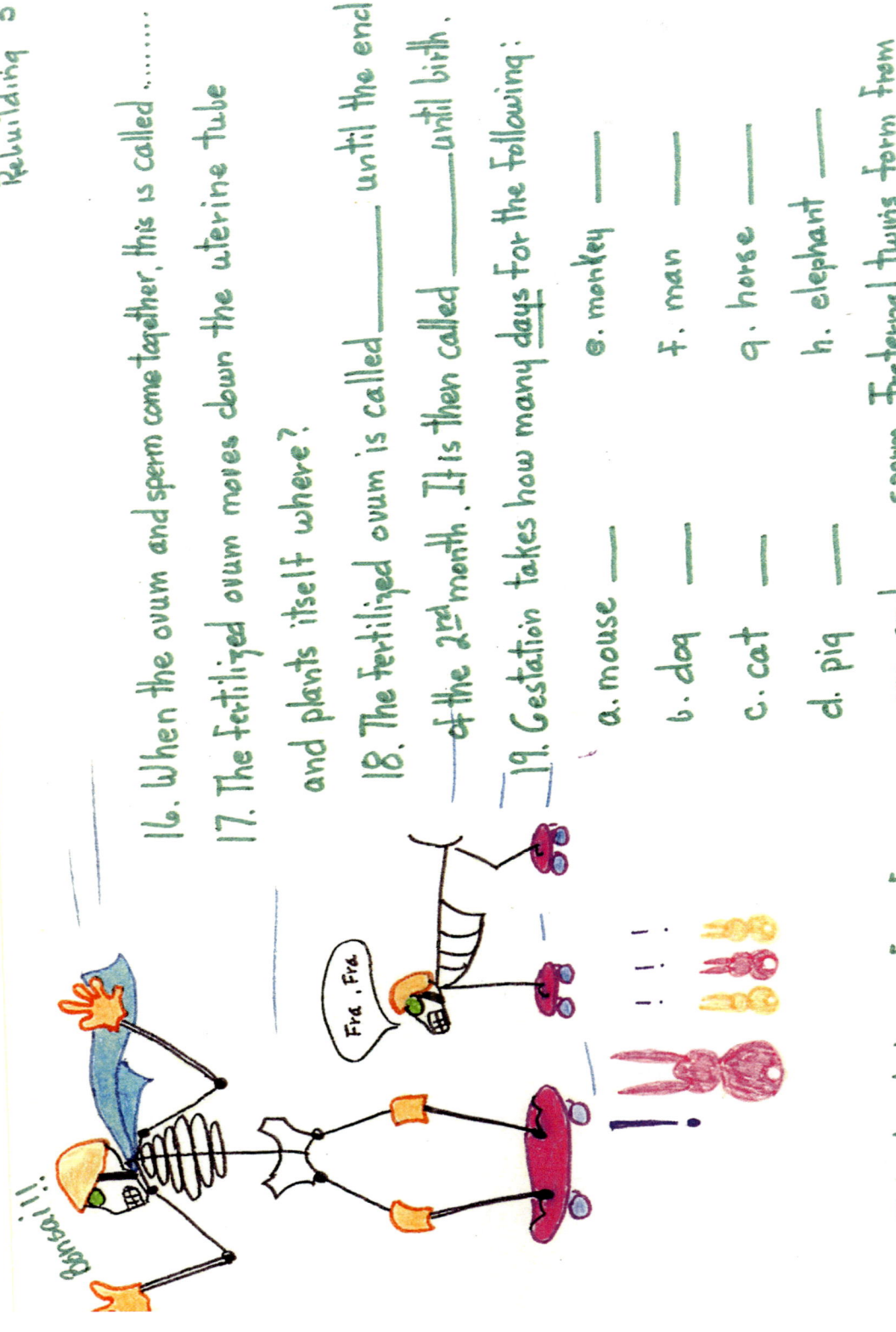

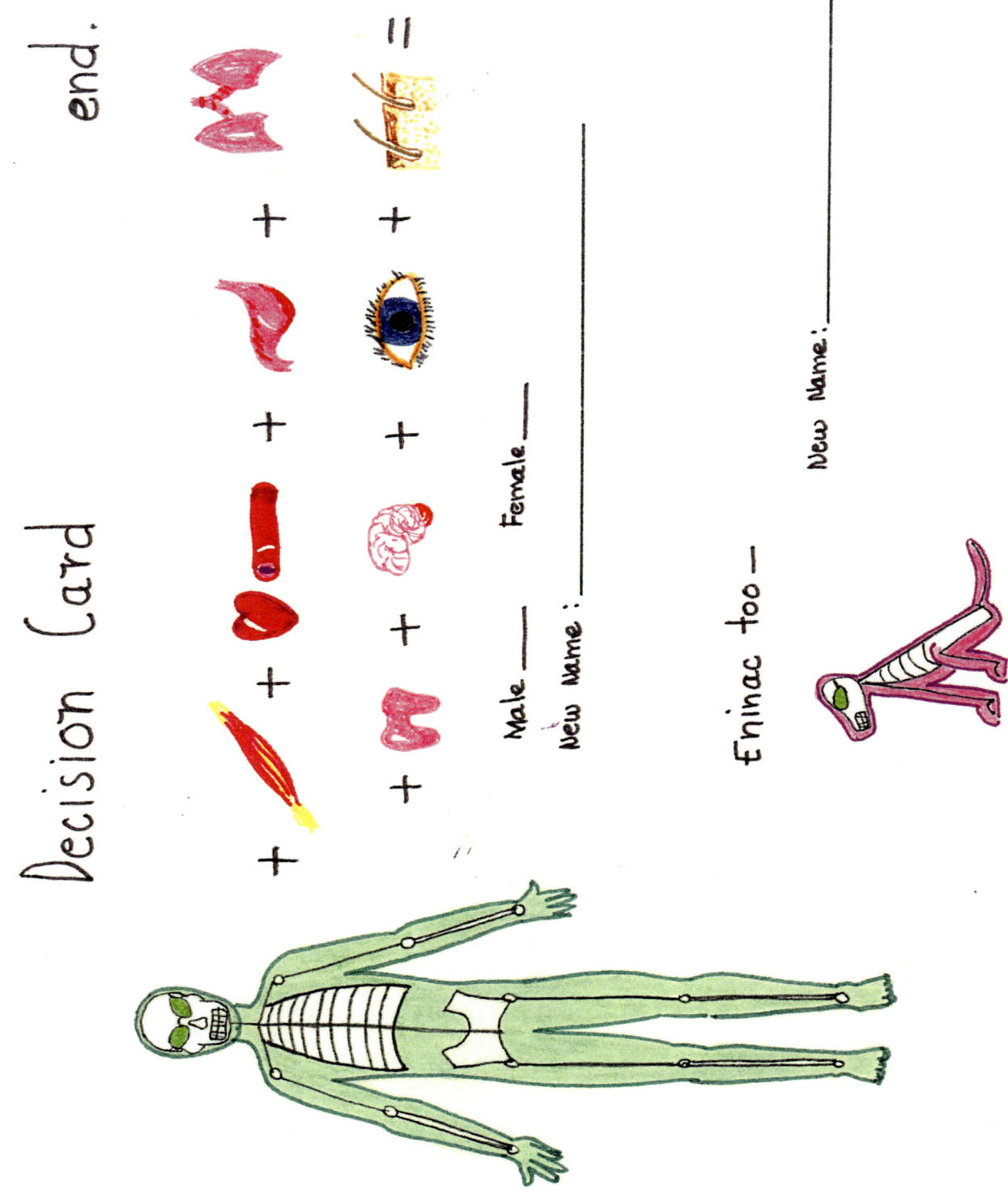

WORKBOOK ANSWERS

| ANSWERS | POINTS |

Unit 1 Skeleton

1. 206	1
2. Support and protection	2
3. Vertebral column	1
4. 33	1
5. Cartilage	1
6. Skull	1
7. Spinal cord	1
8. Ribs, 24, true ribs, false ribs	4
9. 3, 8, 5, 12, 2	5
10. Femur, thigh	2
11. Hinge, no, hinge, knee (elbow)	4
12. Meek, wrist (ankle), hip (shoulder)	3
13. Ligaments	1
14. Synovial	

Unit 2 Siding-Muscle

1. Tendon	1
2. Brain	1
3. Paralysis	1
4. Yes	1
5. Muscle tone	1
6. Food and use	1
7. Heredity	1
8. Shorter	1
9. Flexors, extensors	2
10. Smooth	1
11. lactic acid	1
12. Oxygen	1
13. Smooth	1
14. Champ	1
15. Hemorrhage	1
16. Chemical, thermal, electrical	3
17. Smooth	1

Unite 3 Heart and Circulation

1. No, no	2
2. Pump	1
3. Right Left	2
4. Body, lungs	2
5. Auricle, ventricle	2
6. Coronary circulation	1
7. Ventricle	1
8. Right auricle, pace maker, left auricle, Right ventricle, left ventricle	5
9. RA to RV to lung to LA to LV to Aorta	6
10 Valves closing	1
11. Aorta, vena cava	2
12. Capillaries	1
13. Lungs	1
14. Dies	1
15. Lymph	1
16. Harding of the arteries	1
17. 100,000	1
18. Veins,, arteries	2
19. Valves (vein cups)	1
20. Pace maker (sinatorial node)	1
21. Sinoartrial node	1
22. 72	1
23. Spleen, liver	2
24. 120 over 80	1
25. High	1
26. Blood stream	1

Unite 4 Digestion

1. Mouth, esophagus, stomach, small intestine, large intestine	5
2. 5	1
3. Mouth, stomach, small intestine	3
4. Enzymes	1
5. Mouth	1
6. 1 – 2 quarts	1
7. Peristalsis	1
8. 2 quarts	1
9. Protein, makes pepsin work faster, dissolves minerals, kills bacteria	4
10. Mucus coating	1

11. Pyloric	1
12. 20 Feet	1
13. Musentery	1
14. Small Intestine	1
15. Starch, protein, fats	3
16. Villa, absorb food	2
17. Absorb water	1
18. Crecum	1
19. End of caecum	1
20. A, D	2

Unit 5 Respiration

1. Gills, skin, spiracles, stornata	4
2. Yes	1
3. No	1
4. R, 3, 2, L	4
5. Lack of oxygen	1
6. Respiration	1
7. (b)	1
8. (d)	1
9. Cilia, mucous membrane	2
10. (a)	1
11. Pharynx	1
12. High, 2	2
13. Larynx	1
14. Thicker vocal cords	1
15. Diaphragm	1
16. Medulla	1
17. Rapid breathing	1
18. Hiccups	1
19. Alveoli	1
20. Heart	1
21. Mechanical	1
22. Exhale	1
23. Inflammation of the Larynx	1

Unit 6 Endocrine System

1. Ductless	1
2. Hormones	1
3. Regulate	1
4. Pineal, pituitary, parathyroid, thymus, adrenal, pancreas, ovaries, testes	9
5. Master gland	1
6. a. Adrenal cortex	5
b. Regulates production of eggs and sperm	
c. Thyroid	
d. Growth	
e. Prolactin	
7. Insulin	1
8. Panaceas	1
9. Thyroid	1
10. Adrenal gland	1
11. Digestion	1
12. a. Adrenal	14
b. Thyroid	
c. Testes	
d. Pancreas	
e. Thyroid	
f. Ovaries	
g. Parathyroid	
h. Pituitary	
i. Pituitary	
j. Thymus	
k. Pineal	
l. Pituitary	
m. Pituitary	
n. Thyroid	
13. Problem: Pituitary making body changes	2

Unit 7 Nerves

Central, peripheral, automatic	3
Neurons	1
Electro-chemical	1
Sensory, carries stimuli from sense organs	6
Motor, makes muscles move	
Associative, (connecting) connects between motor & sensory	

Gray	1
Thinnest	1
Farthermost	1
Sensory	1
Cranial or peripheral, spinal	2
Motor	1
Optic	1
Plexus	1
Involuntary	1
Sympathetic & parasympathetic	2
Yes	1
Reflex	1
Para sympathetic	1
Synapse	1
Neutron drawing	5
Dendrite	
Axon	
Cell body	
Synapse	
end brush	

Unit 8 Brain

brain, spinal cord	2
skull, vertebral column	2
meninges	1
cerebrospinal	1
cerebrum	1
cerebral cortex	1
convolutions	1
movement	1
left movement	1
cerebrum	1
cerebellum	1
hypothalamus, pons	2
medulla	1
Cord	1
(1) Cerebrum	7
(2) Thalamus	
(3) Cerebellum	

Unit 8 Brain cont'd
    (4) Pons
    (5) Medulla
    (6) Cord
    (7) Pituitary

16. (1) Memory (thought)   8
    (2) Motor
    (3) Touch
    (4) Sight
    (5) Hearing
    (6) Taste
    (7) Smell
    (8) Speech

17. a. cerebrum   14
    b. cerebrum
    c. thalamus
    d. hypothalamus
    e. midbrain
    f. cerebrum
    g. hypothalamus
    h. pons
    i. medulla
    j. cerebrum
    k. cerebellum
    l. medulla
    m. cerebellum
    n. cerebrum

Unit 9 Senses

None, no, yes, no, grinds glasses	5
Selene	1
Choroid	1
Retina	1
Cornea	1
None (it's a hole)	1
Iris	1
Iris or pupil	1
Lens	1
Accommodation	1

Vitreous	1
Rods, cones, rods light, cones color	4
Fovea	1
Blind spot	1
A 1	
Binocular	1
Lens	1
1. Optic nerve	8
2. Sclera	
3. Choroid	
4. Retina	
5. Iris	
6. Corona	
7. Lens	
8. Vitreous humor	
19. Audiometer	1
20. Otologist	1
21. Outer, middle, inner	3
22. Eardrum	1
23. Eustachian tube	1
24. Semi-circular canals	1
25. no, no air	2
26. Auditory	1
27. yes	1
28. Soccule and utricle	2
29. 1. Eardrum	9
2. Outer ear	
3. Hammer	
4. Semicircular canals	
5. Auditory nerve	
6. Cochlea	
7. Eustachian tube	
8. Stirrup	
9. Anvil	

Unit 10 Reproduction

Female	1
Male	1
Puberty	1
Pituitary	1
Testosterone, yes	1
Secondary sex characteristics	1
Estrogen, yes	2
Ovulation	1
Menstruation	1
28	1
14	1
Sperm	1
Uterus, ovaries	2
Penis, testes	2
Vagina	1
Fertilization or conception	1
Uterus	1
Embryo, fetus	2
Dog, cat, mouse, pig, monkey, men, horse, elephant	8
1, 1, 2, 2	4
Yes	1